The Strange Case of the Missing Myelin
(Decoding Multiple Sclerosis)

Rafael González Maldonado

Title: *The Strange Case of the Missing Myelin*

Subtitle: *(Decoding Multiple Sclerosis)*

Author: *Rafael González Maldonado*

Prologue: Eduardo Varela de Seijas

1st Spanish edition, 1998
1st English edition, 1998
Last reprinting, may 2013.

Traslated to English by : Jean Louise Sanders

Edited by Rafael González Maldonado

NOTICE.
The information in this book is merely general guidance on the various data
and opinions, sometimes contradictory, issued by multiple sources.
It can not be used without prior consultation with your regular doctor.

To María José

"En ti está la delicia como está la crueldad en las espadas"

(J.L. Borges.)

The Strange Case of the Missing Myelin
Rafael González Maldonado

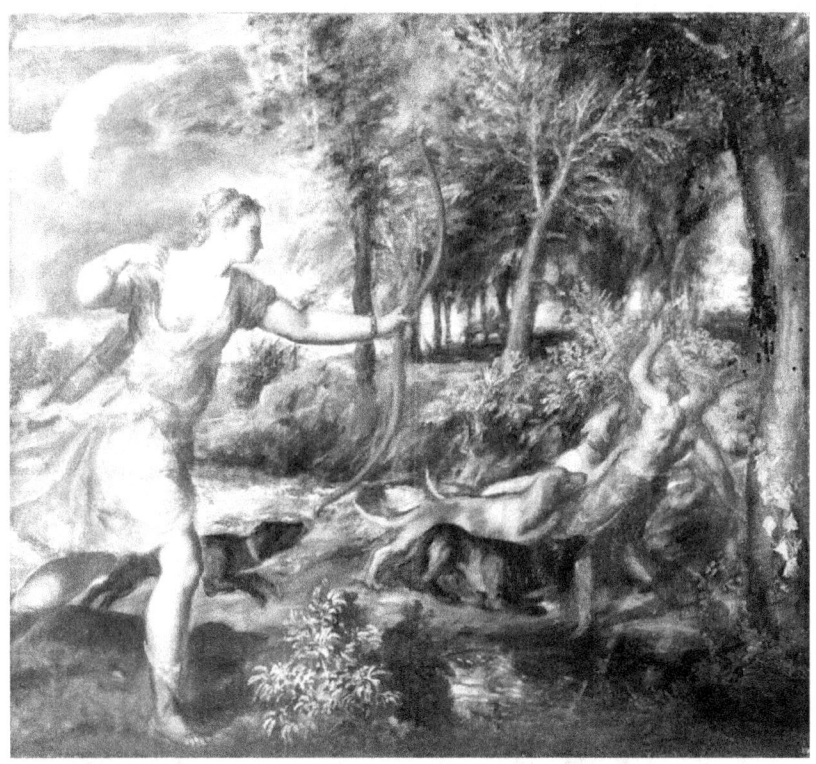

Cover illustration. Acteon and Diane(Tiziano; The National Gallery, London.)

The myth of autoimmunity: *Acteon is devoured by his own hounds, who do not recognize him. In multiple sclerosis, the lymphocytes destroy the myelin because they perceive it as something foreign or strange.*

Prologue

A year ago, the author of this book introduced an original and attractive style of scientific communication with the publication of *The Strange Case of Dr. Parkinson*. Despite all its intrinsic value, it might have gone down as an isolated dot on the scientific biography of Rafael González Maldonado. The publication of the book that you hold in your hands represents another point of interest on that biography. And two points —as we learned in the early years of that archaic form of schooling we received— make a line. In this case, an intellectual path.

I am not going to analyze the scientific background of this work, which constitutes an impressive review of the current situation of multiple sclerosis: its etiopathogeny, physiopathology, clinical presentation, diagnosis and treatment. The bibliography is very complete, carefully chosen and up-to-date, *à la page*, as they say in French.

The wealth in new and established scientific data alone would justify this publication as a book of reference for physicians in general, and an intensive course, of sorts, for many neurologists. But what makes this editorial route original are the language and the resources that the author makes use of in order to communicate alluringly, "charming" the reader into the often arid (for the uninitiated), extense and confusing terrain of neurological pathology. As Hugo Liaño stated in the prologue to *The Strange Case of Dr. Parkinson*, the author has hit upon the philosopher's stone of written communication in the medical field.

Scientific communication is becoming more and more cryptic, in part owing to the enormous increase in the amount of scientific facts and concepts, and the need to condense them in articles and books that can be read in a relatively short time. Yet the abundance of neologisms, latinisms, loanwords, acronyms, conventionalisms, initials and eponyms that saturate today's medical texts make them intelligible only to insiders. Thus, an article on cardiology is barely comprehensible for an endocrinologist or rheumatologist; and this happens in all the specialized fields of medicine. Often the reader has to go back over an article searching for the meaning of initials that clog the text, rending useless the author's intentions of saving time by economizing with words.

Behind the evolution of the cryptic text hides, most likely, a desire for control by a reduced group of persons. The possession of knowledge — considered, rightly, as the key to power— and the control of its diffusion through language have been wielded from primitive societies to modern ones by closed circles that adopt rites and liturgies apt only for the initiated, with the unfailing presence of a high priest, a sanhedrin, and some novices or neophytes.

This has gone on, historically and transculturally, since the time of the Pythagoreans, on through the Masons, and Rosicrucians, up to the secret Melanesian societies studied by R. H. Codrington, or the Hung society in China. These groups use language as their main differential element with respect to the rest of the community, and this language tends to become artificially complex. A steady outpour of books and publications attempt to placate this centrifugal force in the sphere of scientific communication, which would leave a black hole in the layman's knowledge of Science.

Such texts come into being with one of two original sins: either their authors are authentic experts on the topic in question, in which case, usually but unfortunately, the language used is too difficult for the general public to understand; or else, the authors are *aficionados* with only a superficial understanding of the topic, who mistreat and twist scientific reality. In the first case, the language is what suffers; in the second, it is the concept.

As a counterpoint to all this, our century has seen the development of journalistic-commercial communication, with objectives that are diametrically opposed to those mentioned above. In this case what matters, above all, is attracting the attention of the mass-individual, who is blunted by multiple competing stimuli, and then transmitting an idea or concept reduced to elementary terms, with a simple, concise, clear and convincing language that is accessible to a "massive, heterogeneous, anonymous and geographically disperse" public (*C.C. Hopkins, McDougall*).

The neuropsychological foundation of this approach is the conditioned reflex, with its reciprocal game of stimulus and response. The stimulus must be strong and specific enough to attract the attention of the person to whom it is directed. Capturing the attention of the reader is, then, the primary objective of journalistic-commercial communication, and for that reason the textist (a horrendous word used in the world of publicity, but which is useful for distinguishing the publicity writer from the real writer) has no qualms about using tricks, conventionalisms and more or less coarse appeals to the reader's instincts or subconscious underlays.

Where, on the graph of written communication, do we situate the work at hand? Is it scientific exposition or journalistic narrative? It is precisely in the analysis of this junction where the originality and excellence of this book lie.

The Strange Case of the Missing Myelin is, indeed, a scientific work. The volume of information and the rigor with which it is expounded are determinant. It does not fit the usual mold for works of scientific diffusion, yet it does manage to introduce or clarify, with meridian transparency, and for any person interested, whether patient or doctor, the fundamental aspects of the problem and the "state of the art" of the disease.

The Strange Case of the Missing Myelin is not a journalistic narrative, yet it uses language honestly to allure and hold the interest of the reader. The author resorts to a wide range of tools. Just as the Argentinian *gaucho* slinging bolas or the western cowboy and his lasso manage to bring down the wild pony, this author captures one's attention. The enigmatic chapter headings urge the reader on to decipher their meaning. The short paragraphs prevent fatigue. The anecdote, the diaphanous wording so quick to offer an explanation when technical terms come up, the literary quotes and historical or mythological footnotes, all contribute to pleasureful reading. And so the didactic intentions of the author are fulfilled. The profusion of humanistic references is so great that at times we are left wondering whether the humanities are being taught through pathological medicine, or vice versa. In any case, the combination is perfectly suited to its purposes.

The analogy with the myth of Actaeon, King of Tebas, who was devoured by his hounds at the wrathful orders of Diana, strikes me as beautifully appropriate. Were the dogs unable to recognize their master? Or was it because the goddess had covered him with a deerhide that the dogs misdirected their aggressivity? This is precisely the nature of the mystery —to date— that would explain the antigen-antibody interrelation and the lack of recognition of the body's own myelinic antigens (Actaeon) by the misdirected immune system (the dogs). Never was there a more elegant literary portrait of the immunological conflict behind multiple sclerosis. Again we see to what an extent the modern world is inscribed in the classics when someone has the knowledge and sensitivity to point out the correspondence.

The Strange Case of the Missing Myelin augurs the same success as its predecessor. I recommend that physicians in general read it for a clear, comprehensible, pleasant and present-day introduction to multiple sclerosis, and that neurologists derive from it an effective method of communication with their patients. Because, as ANTIPHON said in 474 B.C., the doctor must speak the evil... yet say it well. Our patients, in their distress, will agree that a tangible ignorance is less damaging to the spirit than a ghostly one.

Prof. Eduardo Varela de Seijas[i]

Introduction

The coasts of Sicily are sown with watchtowers against possible invaders. That morning the watchman fell asleep at his post, and the Viking ship arrived before the people of the village could flee. It was a rapid Norse victory.

As they drank, the Vikings divided up their spoils. Gunthar got a silver goblet and two female prisoners. He raped the younger one, and ordered the other woman to prepare him a bath. His tired body was relaxing in the hot water[i] when suddenly he felt a tingling in his legs, just as he had felt the past spring, only this time more intense. At once he noticed that his left hand was growing weak, and he was overcome with anguish: it was that disease, the family curse.

It afflicted his father, Ragner, who had ruled over Thule for the last ten years without being able to get up from his chair. And his sister, who lost her eyesight as a child, and cousin Sigrid of Scotland, who had begun to walk as if she were drunk. The frightened Viking did not know that his neurons were losing myelin, and that his disease would some day be called multiple sclerosis. We still do not know the cause, but, according to the most popular theory at present,[411,412] there is a genetic predisposition that Gunthar and those of his seafaring race were responsible for spreading.

Others believe that multiple sclerosis is triggered by viruses that were transmitted by British soldiers during World War II.[271-273] Still others say that dogs are to blame, or that it has to do with dental fillings. We do know that the disease is prevalent in Northern countries, and that it affects women more than men, especially well-to-do women who live in the city. No Gypsies or Eskimos are known to suffer the disease, and some people take primula oil to prevent it. The evolution of multiple sclerosis is so diverse that we must ask ourselves if it is really one disease or many. Can surgery help? Do those costly new treatments really work?

This book sums up and attempts to pleasantly explain the huge mass of information available about multiple sclerosis. With scientific rigor and a communicative vocation, we shall try to "decipher" the keys to the disease. The reader will find a great number of facts, and, here and there, an odd hypothesis, a classic quotation, or an intuitive suggestion. Because knowledge (like love) needs flavoring.

1. Multiple stories

Multiple sclerosis is considered a young disease, because it affects young adults, and also because it was identified in recent times. Ancient descriptions of the disease are few and unreliable (perhaps the symptoms were somewhat different then). Its frequency is on the rise since the 19th century.[253]

THE NAMES OF THE DISEASE

We may name a disease after its main symptom, as in epilepsy or migraine. Other times an eponym is used, that is, the proper name of the person who defined the disease, such as Alzheimer´s or Parkinson´s disease. But the disease in question here has no characteristic symptom nor eponym,[ii] and even its name varies from one country to another. The French refer to it as sclerosis in plaques; the English call it disseminated sclerosis; and Americans coined the term "multiple sclerosis."

A 14TH CENTURY NUN

The first person believed to have multiple sclerosis was born in Holland in 1380, became a nun, and was canonized as a saint after her death.[336] For 37 years, Saint Lidwina von Schiedham suffered neurological symptoms that grew worse periodically, and that suggested lesions on multiple sites of the nervous system.

IF NOT CHASTE, BE CAUTIOUS

George III of England was not familiar with the readings of Gracián.[iii] He was neither chaste nor cautious, and everyone knew the story of his illegitimate grandchild, August Frederick d'Esté (1794-1848). He was the biological cousin of Queen Victoria, and we know from his diaries[150] that he suffered from multiple sclerosis. He wrote:

(At age twenty-eight:)*"I was returning from a funeral and I went blind. Some time later I recovered the strength and clarity of my eyesight completely."*

(Five years later, in Florence, a relapse:) *"I remained very weak for twenty-one days, falling because my legs were not able to support my body."*

(In 1830, the sexual vigor inherited from his grandfather declines:) *"I had an affaire with a young woman, and found when I lay with her that I had lost my healthy vigour."*

His legs grow weaker and weaker, and by his fiftieth birthday August Frederick D'Este is in a wheelchair. The progression of his tremor is evident in the manuscript, whose final lines are illegible. He died two years later.

THE MAID GETS HIS ATTENTION

For a maid with multiple sclerosis, it was a stroke of luck to be employed at the Charcot household. The "father of classic Neurology" was able to closely observe, over years, the symptoms of the young woman (nystagmus, intention tremor, scanning speech).[57] Yet... he was mistaken about the diagnosis: Charcot said it was a case of tabes. The autopsy was conclusive: there were multiple zones of disseminated sclerosis.

A *DE*-MYELINATING DISEASE

Multiple sclerosis is a demyelinating disease. It alters and destroys myelin, the membrane that covers the long nerve fibers (axons), protecting them, isolating them and enhancing their electrical conductivity.

Myelin is a shiny white substance made up of lipids and proteins. It is produced by the oligodentrocytes,[iv] cells that surround the neurons.

When the myelin is destroyed (demyelination), the axon is bared, unprotected, and does not conduct the nerve impulse properly. That is when the symptoms appear. They will vary, depending on the site of affection in the brain or spinal cord.

OPEN THE BODIES TO SEE THE DISEASE[v]

"No disease exists without site nor cause," proclaimed the doctors of old. They opened dead bodies in search of lesions that would explain the symptoms. And thus, anatomical pathology was born.

The basic lesion in multiple sclerosis is called a plaque.

There is some question as to who first described these plaques. In a marvellous collectible human atlas (published 1829-1842), Cruveilhier[99] referred to zones of firm consistency that formed "stains" or "islets" in a patient with *"paraplegia from grey degeneration of the funiculi of the medulla spinalis."*

But by the time this chapter came out, many doctors had already seen the illustrations by Robert Carswell (1838) of "a peculiar disease of the spinal cord and brain stem with atrophic discoloured zones."[83]

DIAGNOSE THEM WHILE THEY ARE ALIVE

His predecessors talked of autopsies. But the German pathologist and clinician Frerichs, in 1849, made the first diagnosis of a live patient. He said the patient had *Hirnsklerose*.[165] Seven years later, the autopsy proved him right.

The first clear definition of the symptoms of multiple sclerosis came from Jean Marie Charcot, in his famous clinical sessions at the Hospital de la Salpêtrière (1872-1873). He distinguished it from amiotrophic lateral sclerosis, whose only similarity lies in the name. Charcot insisted that patients with multiple sclerosis have an "intention" tremor when they are about to execute a movement, unlike persons with Parkinson´s disease (who have a tremor in repose). He also described the nystagmus (oscillation of the eyes) and the impaired speech (they talk as if they were inebriated).

These three symptoms (nystagmus, tremor and scanning speech) were baptized "Charcot's classic triad." Charcot himself placed only limited importance on them, however, and insisted that a patient could have multiple sclerosis even though one, two, or even all three symptoms were absent. He was right: the triad is rarely present at the onset of the disease, and less than 10% of patients present it eventually. It is no longer considered typical of MS.[391]

THE TOES OF HYSTERICAL WOMEN

Babinski treated patients back in the 19th century, when medical waiting rooms were full of women suffering from hysteria. Multiple sclerosis patients had such varied symptoms that they could be confused with hysteria,[vi] especially when the woman complained of not being able to move her legs.

The sign described by Babinski helped differentiate between the two. In paralysis by lesion of the central nervous system, when the plant of the foot is scratched, the toes (particularly the big toe) extend. Meanwhile, the patients who have no "organic" illness (only hysteria) would have the normal flexion reflex, that is, curling their toes downward.

AT FIRST IT WAS HYSTERICS

And so, at first doctors mistook multiple sclerosis for hysteria, but Babinski learned to differentiate. Well now studies have turned the tables, and once again mix psychiatrics with neurology. Patients with multiple sclerosis present a "hysterical reaction" before relapses (or "flare-ups"), and this type of behavior has its roots in infancy. "Hysterical" children are more likely to have multiple sclerosis when they reach adulthood (see Chapter 6).

A PROTEAN DISEASE

Protean [vii] means variable, having many forms, and it is a key descriptor for multiple sclerosis. Indeed, the diversity in its mode of presentation and its evolution are characteristic. Depending on which zones are demyelinated, sensitive or motor symptoms will appear, with alterations in balance, or vision. Days or years may elapse between one "flare-up" or exacerbation (appearance of new symptoms) and the next.

The lesions are disseminated throughout the central nervous system and differ in size, location, and date of appearance. Each patient evolves at his own pace, and response to treatment is also peculiar. In other words, what characterizes multiple sclerosis is the unity of its diversity. [viii]

THEY GET ILL BECAUSE THEY DON´T SWEAT

Multiple sclerosis is produced because patients do not sweat enough. This was an early explanation of the disease, offered by Cruveilhier.[98]

The list of possible causes[326] continues to grow, demonstrating that we really don´t understand what is going on: mercury fillings, cold, dogs, ticks, or all sorts of germs have been blamed.

Just like fashions come and go, metabolic hyotheses, circulatory causes, infectious or immunological causes and their respective treatments have all been in vogue at some point in time.

When it was thought that the cause was a metabolic disorder, digestive enzymes, vitamins or antidiabetic medications were used for treatment. Later, circulatory problems were hailed as the cause, and vasodilators and anticoagulants were used.

The infectious theory promoted the use of antibiotics, antimicotics and antiviral drugs. Those that suspected an immunological disorder prescribed vaccines, or went so far as to remove the patient´s thymus. Or worse. The book by Sibley[490] describes many fruitless treatments, some completely absurd, of purely historical interest.

A CATALONIAN IN PARIS

Half a century ago, three Soviet scientists[ix] boastfully published: *"We have identified the multiple sclerosis virus."*.

Our prestigious Dr. Barraquer i Bordás was so intrigued that he traveled to Paris to discuss the matter with Professor Mollaret, an expert in infectious diseases.

The tale, as told by our Catalonian compatriot[28] does not go into details about whether it was on a stroll beside the Seine or along the Champs de l'Elysées[ii] when the wise Frenchman revealed what he knew: *"Pay no attention, Luis; what those Russians have discovered is the attenuated rabies virus."*

CRYING AT THE PODIUM

Such refutations are more scalding when they are live and direct. Biomedical researcher Kathleen Chevassut was so sure of having isolated the microbe causing multiple sclerosis that she baptized it: *Spherula insulares*. Hopeful gallantry and a lack of rigor on the part of some illustrious scientists led them to believe she was right.

The optimistic researcher stood up to defend her "discovery" at an important medical meeting. A hard-headed male (E. Arnold Carmichael was not in the best of moods) rebuffed her cruelly and categorically, and Ms Chevassut ran out crying, so devastated that she abandoned research from that moment on .

FROM THOSE SORROWS, THESE PLAQUES

It was Charcot, too, who said that sorrow might be associated with the disease (see Chapter 5, "The mind, moods and personality"). And even before him, Frerichs had made the same observation. Recent studies agree: a divorce, losing one's job, the death of a family member, economic hard times and other negative or stressful circumstances can trigger exacerbations; they may even influence the appearance of the disease.[188-190,253,507,542,543]

It is known that stress affects the immunological system.[77] And after all, its alteration is what brings on multiple sclerosis.

THE NYMPH, THE POET...

Besides the Dutch nun, the cousin of Queen Victoria and Charcot's housemaid, there are other well-known figures who suffered from multiple sclerosis.

Nymphomania was described, of course, by Sigmund Freud. The nymphomaniac was a young woman with an excessive sexual desire. That was the key to diagnosing her multiple sclerosis ¿??? (Shaw mentions it in his//her biography) ¿??? The suicidal person, a literary figure, is depicted in the novel *Shogun* [79] in all his despair when faced with the debilitating disease. ¿???

Two German poets were also afflicted: Eduard Mörike (1804-1875)[253] and Heinrich Heine (1797-1856). Heine is the better known of the two, a hybrid poet combining romanticism and incipient realism[x] who was paralyzed in the later years of his life.[238,245]

ILL DOCTORS

Studying medicine does not prevent multiple sclerosis. In 1843, a medical alumnus of the University of Pennsylvania, Dr. Pennock, began to complain of clumsiness and a tingling sensation in his left leg, and later in his right.[xi] The incapacity increased over the years: his arms grew weak, walking became difficult, and he had problems urinating.

The good doctor died in 1867. He had made the observation, however, that hot water worsened his condition (see Chapter 8 for an explanation of the caldarium test).

Internet has focused the spotlight on one doctor with multiple sclerosis who does not wish to reveal his identity. He signs in as Dr.Gmarc46, and his web pages offer a personal view of the disease that is particularly insightful because of his dual condition as doctor and patient.

He is extremely well informed about the latest research in the area, as well as about home-made remedies. He speaks from experience, sprinkled with irony or skepticism at times, but always rich and enriching. Don't miss it: get on your PC and track him down at http://aspin.asu.edu.

PROFUSE BUT NOT ECUMENICAL[xii]

Multiple sclerosis is a profuse disease (widespread and frequent) but not ecumenical (it does not occur everywhere). Around the world there are over a million sufferers; however, in some countries there are many, and in others only very rare cases. In the U.S. there are 400,000 MS patients,[15,514] whereas in Ethiopia there are practically none.

Epidemiological studies speak to us of the number of "new" cases that appear each year (incidence) and of the total number of cases at a given time (prevalence). In a city of 100,000 inhabitants, each year two new cases of multiple sclerosis are diagnosed (we say, then, that it has an incidence of 2 per 100,000).

But to these new cases we obviously must add the cases from previous years; thus, at a given time our theoretical city of 100,000 inhabitants has many more persons affected by the disease, approximately 55 (that is, a prevalence of 55 per 100,000). In our small Spanish province of Granada (population 800,000) there would be some 440 cases.

Prevalence in Europe and the United States ranges from 15 to 145 per 100,000, depending on the country.[181] In other parts of the world the figures are much lower.

MULTIPLE SCLEROSIS IN SPAIN

The early epidemiological studies of MS carried out in Spain had considerable methodological deficiencies, for which reason the real significance of the disease in our country has only recently become apparent. The pioneer in this field is Oscar Fernández,[138,143,144] who focused much of his research on a sanitary district in the province of Malaga.

More epidemiological studies of multiple sclerosis followed, in the health districts of Alcoy,[318,323] Asturias,[528,529] Navarra,[16] Teruel,[347] and other areas of Spain. Altogether, Spain represents a zone of intermediate risk: incidence is 2 per 100,000 (800 Spaniards come down with symptoms of MS each year); and prevalence is 55 per 100,000 (at present, there are 25.000 persons in Spain with multiple sclerosis).

JUST A FEW LEARNED BOOKS SUFFICE[xiii]

There are many books about multiple sclerosis. Some are written for specialists, some for the general public (in England and the U.S. you can even find them in supermarkets). Let us mention just a few, ones that will be of real interest. Among the "scientific" books that are up-to-date, we recommend the one by Paty and Ebers[391] and the one by Kesselring.[253] In Spanish, the most complete book specifically about MS is the one by Óscar Fernández.[141,142] These are books for neurologists or for physicians with a special interest in the disease.

The most interesting books for the layman are in English: for example, *Learning to Live with Multiple Sclerosis,*[420] *Coping with Multiple Sclerosis,*[46] and *Diets to Help Multiple Sclerosis.*[194] There are also books with a sound scientific basis that are relatively easy to read: *Multiple Sclerosis, Fact Book*[290] and *Therapeutic Claims in Multiple Sclerosis.*[490]

Finally, for patients, family members or doctors who want a thorough introduction to multiple sclerosis, there is a rather strange publication that defies classification: the book you are holding.

2. What is multiple sclerosis?

Multiple sclerosis is an inflammatory disease of the central nervous system (cerbrum, cerebellum, brain stem and spinal cord). The myelin in the white matter[i] is destroyed. Myelin is an insulating material that surrounds the long nerve fibers (axons) and helps transmit electrical impulses. When myelin is lost, the nerve conducts impulses poorly, and the symptoms of the disease appear.

The lesiones seen in MS are called "plaques," and they differ from one individual to the next. They may be small or large; some are "active" and some are "chronic." They can appear at any time, usually in the form of "flare-ups" or relapses (when the patient´s symptoms are exacerbated), followed by periods of recovery or remission.

Patients are born with a predisposition to "auto-immune" type reactions. During childhood they have contact with some external factor (possibly a virus) that makes them develop the autoimmune response which, years later, will produce the inflammation and demyelination of the brain or spinal cord.

MULTIPLE DISSEMINATED PLAQUES

In multiple sclerosis, the lesions are multiple, they form plaques, and they are disseminated, scattered diffusely throughout the brain and the spinal cord. The "plaque" is a zone of white matter in which the myelin sheath of the axons is missing (demyelination). As a result, the axons appear somewhat modified, yet relatively well preserved.

The plaques are usually small, less than a centimeter in diameter, except when they are grouped together or "coalesce," which is the general tendency.

In most cases they surround small veins (perivenular disposition) and they are more frequent around the ventricles (periventricular predisposition). Outside the brain, the plaques damage the optic nerves, the brain stem, and the cervical spinal cord.

DELENDA EST MIELINA[ii]

"May the myelin be destroyed!" is the command given within the altered immunological system of patients with multiple sclerosis.

Myelin is a substance that surrounds and protects nerve fibers, and is made up of proteins and lipids. In multiple sclerosis, the immunological system is damaged and does not recognize some of the components of the myelin. It considers them foreign enemies, and orders the immune cells (lymphocytes and macrophages) to attack the myelin.

The result is an inflammatory and immune response similar to that produced when a bacteria is introduced in the organism; only that lymphocytes and macrophages attack the body's own myelin, because they mistake it for a virus. The "demyelinated" lesions produced are the cause of the symptoms that will appear.

I ACCUSE THE T LYMPHOCYTES

They are called T lymphocytes (or simply T cells) because they are produced in the Thymus.[iii] They are the executioners, the ones that do the damage. They provoke the inflammation and the demyelination, the destruction of the myelin sheath.

The T lymphocytes are responsible not only for initiating the inflammatory reaction but also for amplifying it, and its conclusion possibly depends on them as well. In addition, the T lymphocytes are involved in the production of cytokines, which are very important mediators in the immunological reaction.[555]

THE BITTER ROLE OF CHROMOSOME 6

The confused state of the T lymphocytes can be traced back to chromosome 6, which regulates immunity. It plays the role of minister of defense, deciding how the body is going to react to acts of aggression. Within chromosome 6 commands are given to destroy the bacteria that attack our system, or the dust that bothers our bronchia.

Chromosome 6 is responsible or our defenses, but sometimes, for instance with allergies, it so happens that the "counterattack" to isolate the pollen or the toxin in a beesting produces so much inflammation that the remedy is worse than the disease.

Other times it simply errs, as is the case with "autoimmune" diseases: the body wages a battle against itself, attacking proteins that it doesn't recognize as its own, mistaking them for enemies. In multiple sclerosis, myelin is the victim.[iv]

The susceptibility to multiple sclerosis resides in a specific section of the chromosome called the HLA (human lymphocyte antigens).[30,458]

It is there where the genes that determine the behavior of our immunological system gather to finally order the attack on the body's nerve tissue. An acerb patrimony, indeed![v]

MYELIN, LYMPHOCYTES, AND ACTEON´S HOUNDS

Actaeon, a classic *voyeur*, entertained himself by watching naked Diana (Artemis for the Greeks) bathe in the river. When he was found out, the goddess of the hunt angrily issued the sentence that he no longer be recognized by his own hounds (who had always protected him). Hence, the "confused" animals attacked and devoured their master. This ancient myth tells the story of what lymphocytes do when they do not recognize their own myelin, and "devour" it. The cause of the confusion is chromosome 6, in the role of Diana.

BREAKING BARRIERS

They say[453] that the plaques appear in places where certain traumatisms have broken the blood-brain barrier.[vi] For this reason, the optic nerves are affected (they are very mobile, constantly exposed to minor traumatisms), or the spinal cord (at the points of junction with the notched ligaments) and the zones surrounding the ventricles (the sharp angles favor a "cutting" distension).

These are precisely the sites where plaques appear most frequently, which is why some specialists invoke the "traumatic" or mechanical factor we have just described. The hypothesis was put forth by Lord Brian///Brain ¿?? and Marcia Wilkinson thirty years ago: in the autopsy of a patient with multiple sclerosis and cervical arthrosis, the plaques coincided exactly with the zones where the altered vertebral discs had put pressure on the spinal cord.

SALMON-COLORED PLAQUES

When exacerbations occur, acute plaques appear, with a pinkish salmon color. The lesioned zone has irregular edges, and inflammation is noteworthy, with infiltrated cells (T lymphocytes, macrophages) and remains of the myelin that is being digested. Oligodendrocytes (the cells that make up the myelin) are under attack and their number diminishes, while the astrocytes increase in number (astrocytosis) when exacerbations occur.

Proportionately, there is no major change in the nerve axons. For this reason –in many patients—the lesions are reversible at first, and the symptoms may later improve or disappear.[104]

GRAY, LIKE THE ASHES OF THE PHOENIX

The chronic plaques are gray in color. They are the oldest lesions, the ones described by the early anatomists. Their edges are better defined, clearly cut, and and they bear little evidence now of inflammatory activity or cellular remnants. The oligodendrocytes are degenerated, the myelin is missing. The axons are damaged and appear bare amid an overgrowth of tiny glial fibers (gliosis).[354]

This chronic plaque looks like a "wasteland." It is a silent lesion, apparenly dead or dormant, but in some relapses it may reactivate —like the Phoenix,[i] rising up from its ashes. Then no new symptoms are observed, but the previous problems get worse or more extensive.

THE SEQUELAE DEPEND ON THE AXON

After all these years talking about myelin, it turns out that what really matters in terms of aftereffects (sequelae) is whether the axon is damaged. When a nerve zone loses myelin it ceases to function, but if the axon is not broken, it recovers (for example, in optic neuritis, the lost vision is usually recovered). The sequelae or future incapacities depend, in the final analysis, on the number of axons destroyed. The current trend in research is to study the mechanism through which axons are destroyed and the factors involved in their evolution.[521]

IN A NUTSHELL

Multiple sclerosis, then, is produced in individuals with a genetic predisposition (susceptible from birth on) and in whom an abnormal immunological reaction (an altered "defense" of the organism) is set off as a result of contact with certain infectious agents (virus or other).

Consequently, the lymphocytes (and other elements) attack the myelin of the body's own nerve fibers (in the spinal cord or brain). When the myelin is destroyed, a series of symptoms appear: paralysis, sensitive alterations, lack of coordination, or others. If the lesion is extensive and axons are lost, there will be sequelae; if not, recovery is likely.

Generally speaking, the onset of the disease is acute (brief), slight at first, and possibly reversible. Later, over some years, it will evolve in the form of exacerbations that lead to an accumulation of incapacities.

Eventually the relapses increase in frequency and may reach the point of a chronic form, in which the lesions (and therefore the symptoms) advance slowly but steadily.

DEMYELINATIONS THAT ARE NOT MS

Multiple sclerosis is the best known and most frequent demyelinating disease, but it is not the only one. In the central nervous system (and the peripheral one) there are other possible alterations of the myelin.

They are very rare, and most general physicians never come across a case in their professional career. The only thing they have in common with multiple sclerosis is the fact that the myelin is disturbed, but through different mechanisms.

We mention them here briefly: central pontine myelinolysis (localized loss of myelin in the pons, or protuberance in some sodium imbalances), progressive multifocal leukoencephalopathy (in patients with AIDS, certian opportunistic viruses infect the oligodendrocytes), acute disseminated encephalomyelitis (of the three, the most similar condition, in which an autoimmune reaction against the myelin is triggered by infection or vaccination).[i]

OPTIC NEURITIS AS THE HERALD

Some persons suddenly lose their eyesight because the myelin covering the optic nerve is affected. This is a "demyelinating" optic neuritis which is usually transitory and unaccompanied by other neurological symptoms, and vision returns after a few days or weeks. This good recovery is precisely what distinguishes it from other types of optic neuritis, such as ischemic optic neuritis, which has a much poorer prognosis.[544]

Optic neuritis may affect one or both sides, and it used to be considered an autonomous entity, but now we know that half of these patients will suffer from multiple sclerosis later on. Even among those who have no other symptoms, magnetic resonance imaging may show that the brain and spinal cord have demyelinating lesions as well. It has become clearer to doctors that an optic neuritis is a "frustrated" multiple sclerosis, or its herald,[vii] the first manifestation or announcement of the disease.[163]

THE FRUSTRATED TRANSVERSE MYELITIS

Transverse myelitis can be considered another incomplete or "frustrated" multiple sclerosis. The demylination takes place in the spinal cord, only once, in theory at least. Many times it comes as the first warning: 80% of the patients with transverse myelitis eventually develop a true multiple sclerosis.[157]

COUSIN GUILLAIN-BARRÉ

The Guillain-Barré syndrome (otherwise known as acute idiopathic polyneuritis) is related to multiple sclerosis. It has a similar demyelinating mechanism, only instead of affecting the brain or spinal cord, the peripheral nerves of the extremities are damaged. Guillain-Barré is to the peripheral nervous system what multiple sclerosis is to the central nervous system.

They may constitute two different forms of reacting to similar stimuli through a similar mechanism, their differences owing to the blood-brain barrier (present in the brain and spinal cord, but not in the nerves).

A VIRTUAL MODEL OF SCLEROSIS

Virtual models have many applications. Years ago, in order to design an automobile or appraise an architectural project, a scale model was built. Today we use computers to come up with the "virtual model": a representation of whatever it is we want to study, or to test.

In studying disease, we need to carry out experiments, some entailing health risks, and patients cannot be used.

Therefore, in order that research might advance, it is vital to obtain experimental animals who can provide an "example of the disease" as close as possible to the disease we wish to study in humans.

We already have animal models for Parkinson's disease, for Alzheimer's, and for other diseases. The virtual model for multiple sclerosis in animals is called experimental allergic encephalitis.[88,304]

EXPERIMENTING WITH ALLERGIC ENCEPHALITIS

If we inject nerve tissue into a mouse, an "allergic" reaction (immunopathology) occurs, producing a destruction of the myelin in the brain and spinal cord that closely resembles multiple sclerosis. Now we can study the effects of a number of factors that contribute to experimental encephalitis (age, sex, etc.) and observe the benefits (or drawbacks) of the different treatments.[317]

There are, in fact, different models of "experimental encephalitis," depending n the substance injected into the animal, the dose, and the type of animal used. Some models are more similar to the relapsing-remitting form of MS, others to the monophasic forms (with only one flare-up) and other variations. Each model can prove useful for a different purpose.

THE VIRUS THAT DEMYELINATES MICE

Experimental allergic encephalitis did not exist until man invented it. But some mice spontaneously suffer from a demyelinating disease that is also quite similar to multiple sclerosis. It was discovered unexpectedly by Theiler, who noticed that the hindlegs of some of his mice were paralyzed. He investigated, and found out that a virus was the cause (Theiler's mouse encephalomyelitis virus).[518]

The infected mice began with symptoms similar to those of poliomyelitis (early stage); then they suffered a sort of multiple sclerosis (late stage) with demyelination of the spinal cord as the infection continued and became chronic.

Thus, we find ourselves face to face with a spontaneous demyelination that can be provoked in lab animals by inoculating them with a virus, and our experimental results can be extrapolated to learn more about multiple sclerosis in humans.[352,525]

MOSQUITOS IN THE JUNGLES OF UGANDA

It takes real daring and perseverance to go to the jungles of Uganda,[viii] catch mosquitos, check to see if they are infected with the virus we are looking for, extract and culture the virus, and then inject it into a mouse.

This virus would produce, in the mouse, a disease causing a demyelinating type of cerebral lesion.

NOT CONTAGIOUS, BUT TRANSMITTED

If multiple sclerosis were contagious, there would be numerous cases of spouses contracting the disease, but this does not happen. However, that does not mean that we cannot transmit the disease experimentally: if we have sensitized a lab animal with the proper antigen, its blood serum (to be more exact, the T lymphocytes in the blood) can produce demyelination in a second animal to which it is transfused.

HEALTHY SICK PEOPLE

Aside from the problems deriving from demyelination, MS patients ejnoy good health. They fight off local and systemic infections well, be they from bacteria or fungi. They even suffer fewer viral illnesses than the rest of the population.[491] They do not run an increased risk of cancer or of other autommune diseases. In other words, we cannot say that they have a generalized immune disorder.[117]

In multiple sclerosis the autoimmune activation is specific and limited. And although we have been searching and researching for decades, we still are not able to define the defect. In contrast, there are other autoimmune diseases, such as myasthenia gravis, for which we have identified the target (the acetycholine receptors of the muscle cells). Once the autoantibodies against those receptors are detected and measured, the evolution of the disease can be better assessed.

3. Multiple sclerosis is genetic

In multiple sclerosis there is an immunological disorder that may be from birth or acquired. It is most likely that the mechanism is of a mixed nature: one is born with a genetic susceptibility, and something in the atmosphere (a virus, a toxin, or something else) encountered during childhood or adolescence facilitates the appearance of the disease years later. Depending on the relative importance given to these two factors, there are hypotheses with a genetic basis (which we will see in this chapter) and others that advocate the environmental circumstances (to be explained in Chapter 4).

EPIDEMIOLOGISTS CAN HELP

Multiple sclerosis is "idiopathic," meaning simply that we do not yet know its cause (its etiology). What is known is that its pathogeny (the mechanism of production) has an autoimmune base. We just don´t understand what triggers it.

When we do not know what causes a disease, we resort to epidemiology.

We take time to study, and to draw conclusions from, the mode of distribution of the disease with regards to factors such as age or sex (Is it more frequent among the young or old? Women or men?). Or we see if it predominates in certain geographic areas or socio-cultural levels (Does it affect northerners or southerners more often? Europeans or Africans? Coastal populations or inland ones?).

Some epidemiologists may look at ethnic distinctions (certain diseases are known to be more prevalent among Jews, or Blacks, or Caucasians) or certain individual characteristics (nutrition, educational level, cigarette smoking, etc.).

YOUNG NORDIC WOMAN

The prototype of the multiple sclerosis patient would be a white woman, preferentially of Nordic origin, and young (age 25-30), who lives in the city in the middle-to-upper socioeconomic level.[248,274]

The immune system is conditioned by genetic, sexual and hormonal differences.[116] Clearly, this disease predominates in the young woman of childbearing age, and it varies from one country to another. One out of every one thousand Italian women suffers from multiple sclerosis.[187] Yet if we focus on English women aged 33-44, there are four MS patients per one thousand inhabitants;[488] and even more if we look in Scotland or Scandinavia.

GYPSIES AND ESKIMOS, SAFE AND SOUND

They are protected from the disease. It is extremely rare to come across a case of MS among these peoples, regardless of their land of residence. There seems to be a natural immunity to the disease among Gypsies (above all, those from Hungary), Eskimos, and some large African families, such as the Bantu.

Orientals also show some resistance: only one in every 115,000 Chinese suffers from multiple sclerosis.[560] Something similar is observed among the Japanese, even those living far away: in Seattle, Washington, there is a high incidence of multiple sclerosis, yet no cases were found within the Japanese community there.

In New Zealand and Australia there are many MS patients, but the Maori and aborigines are almost never affected.[131,202,334,493]

The Basques of northern Spain have a lower mortality than the rest of the Spanish population. The importance of the genetic factor can hardly be denied.

SICILY 10, MALTA 1

It's not the score of a soccer match, but rather an example of poetic license used to illustrate genetic differences. Sicily and Malta are neighboring islands with similar lifestyles, yet there are ten Sicilians with multiple sclerosis for every Maltese patient.[447,472,533]

The explanation is in the genes. Most of Malta's inhabitants are of Semetic origin; whereas Sicily, like other places in southern Italy, was subjected to a number of colonizations and genetic blendings, including the Viking invasions.

SARDINIA AND THE SONS OF HERCULES

The island of Sardinia holds more than double the number of MS patients than the rest of Italy.[447] Sardinians have a homogenous genetic structure that is completely different from that of the inhabitants of the nearby islands (such as Sicily), or other Italians or Europeans. This fact comes down to us through history and even through mythology.

In the bronze Age, Sardinia was colonized by a strange people of unknown name and origin. They erected eight thousand *nuragas* or stone towers, scattered over the mountains and at the edges of plateaus, possibly to watch over the coasts where invaders often tried to land.[i]

Mythology offers the following evidence of their very special genetic origin: Sardinia was colonized by forty of the children of Hercules, known as the Thespidians.[ii].

THE MYELIN THAT DID NOT MATURE

A century ago a new theory came along affirming that MS patients have a constitutional peculiarity, from birth. Autopsies revealed a lack of maturity of the myelin; in some ways, it was like the myelin of a six-year-old child.

This poorly developed (or poorly conserved?) myelin would be more vulnerable to degradation by a combination of the factors often associated with multiple sclerosis (genetics, the environment, infections and immunological factors).[359,474]

IMMUNOLOGICAL TEMPERAMENT

Chromosome 6 contains the code for the body´s self-defense, the way it reacts when faced with an "enemy" (or what it considers to be an enemy).

As we saw earlier, this chromosone holds the key to our means of defense, our reactions to real or imagined aggressors, and it is unique to an individual. As in psychology, each person reacts differently in the face of adversity, depending on temperament or character. Well then, our immunological "temperament" is determined by the organization of the aminoacid sequences within chromosome 6, specifically, those known as HLA.[iii]

At birth we have a special configuration of these aminoacids, our HLA genotype. The genetic predisposition to multiple sclerosis has been associated with the sites (loci) denominated DR2, and it seems probable that they are mediated by the so-called type-II MHC (major histocompatibility complex).[378]

A RACIST EUROPE

The incidence of multiple sclerosis in European nations varies sharply. Neither climate, nor latitude, nor other environmental causes can justify the variation. The factors are so complex that we find important variations even within a single country. If a comparative study were carried out, ethnicity (racial differences) would be the only datum able to shed some light on the distribution of the disease over the European continent[446]

FOUR PROMISCUOUS NATIONS[iv]

The Israelis, the Palestinians, the Jordanians and the Kuwaitis all live near each other, perhaps too near. For sociopolitical reasons, these four peoples have been mixed together in a small geographical section of the world. And this is important for the epidemiologist.

How does multiple sclerosis behave here? Does the region offer any clues as to a genetic or environmental origin?

They all share a common environment. The greatest similarity in genes is between the Palestinians and Jordanians, who have similar hereditary markers; the Kuwaitis are of a different genetic makeup. Even more distant, both in race and culture, are the Israelis. Let's summarize the risk each group runs of suffering multiple sclerosis: for each Kuwaiti patient there are two Jordanians and four Palestinians.[7-9] The Israelis are affected little, even less than the Kuwaitis.[247,293]

Ethnic features outweigh the environmental ones.

VÍKINGAR FER∂U∂UST MIKI∂

The heading is in the original Viking language,[v] and means "The Vikings traveled far and wide." That is how they extended multiple sclerosis. The disease originated in their race, and they spread it like a family curse all over the many lands that they attacked and colonized. This interesting hypothesis was proposed by Poser in 1995, in a prestigious medical journal.[vi]

In effect, the geographic distribution of multiple sclerosis coincides with the parts of the world that were invaded by the Vikings (Scandinavia, Iceland, the British Isles)[vii] and with the areas of emigration of their Anglo-Saxon descendants (the United States, Canada, Australia and New Zealand).

The Vikings journeyed nearly all over Europe, including Normandy, Galicia, Sicily and southern Italy. They also went as far as Russia, following rivers down to the Caucasus, the Black Sea and the Caspian Sea. They even fought against the Byzantines. Their custom of taking slaves, of keeping the women and children for a time and then selling them, might have played a part in the genetic dissemination of the disease.[411,412] "The curse of Odin"[viii] would appear to still be with us today. At least it is feasible from a genetic viewpoint.

THE RELIGIOUS LEANINGS OF HERPES ZOSTER

In areas with many cases of multiple sclerosis there are also more cases of varicella (better known as chickenpox), which is caused by the herpes zoster virus. We do not have an explanation, but for some reason herpes zoster, varicella, and multiple sclerosis are less frequent among the Hutterite religious sect.[ix] In general, these devoted Anabaptists have a more efficient immune system than their Canadian and American neighbors.[449]

On the other hand, a greater incidence of multiple sclerosis and other autoimmune diseases has been observed for another religious group, the Mennonites now settled in Canada, but of German-Dutch origin. Religious motives can lead to intermarriages within a community and consanguinity. The epidemiologist takes advantage of this circumstance to obtain valuable data when he conducts research on a disease with a hereditary component.[237]

AS IN WOMAN, SO IN THE RAT

Most autoimmune diseases affect women more than men. For instance, rheumatoid arthritis, myesthenia, Sjögren's syndrome, thyroiditis, and lupus erythematosus.[117] The same is true in the animal kingdom: it is easier to produce experimental allergic encephalomyelitis and murine diabetes[537] in female rabbits and lab rats or the females of other species used in laboratory experiments.[537]

Women and female animals have a greater tendency to develop immune self-aggression, their own defenses turning against them. Yet it has nothing to do with masochism.

AS IN MAN, SO IN THE MOUSE

Males have a reduced chance of suffering multiple sclerosis. In the males of other species this disease does not occur spontaneously; but parallels can be drawn with its laboratory equivalent, experimental allergic encephalitis. It is very difficult to induce EAE in young male animals, whereas females are vulnerable.[37]

The number of males with multiple sclerosis is half that of women[x] and their symptoms start later on in life (on the average, three years later). However, more men show a chronic-progressive evolution, a more invalidating form of the disease.[545]

FROM MOTHER TO DAUGHTER

Multiple sclerosis is not inherited or passed down by the Mendelian models we are familiar with. There is something in the environment that must favor it, though no one questions the significance of the genetic factor.

In an intermediate risk zone, the possibility of a person coming down with multiple sclerosis is one in 1,000 if there are no relatives afflicted. When more than one family member is affected, the greatest likelihood is that it is the mother and daughter; what is least likely is to see both the father and son with MS.

If the mother has multiple sclerosis, her daughter runs a one in fifty chance of eventually being affected, whereas the son's chances are much slimmer.

MS PATIENTS HAVE LOTS OF DAUGHTERS

A father with multiple sclerosis is unlikely to have a son with the disease (a chance of one in one hundred), but his daughter is at a greater risk.[459] The fact is, men with multiple sclerosis have more daughters than sons, at least in France,[xi] where this survey was done.[535]

SIBLINGS AND TWINS

We can assess the genetic factor of a disease by studying how it behaves in twins.[210] In order to see how much inheritance and the environment may influence the course of multiple sclerosis, we observe whether or not it coincides in twins, in siblings, in half-brothers/sisters, and in adopted children.[378]

The siblings of an MS patient have a probability of one in 35, the same figure as for bizygotic (fraternal) twins. But if a monozygotic (identical) twin has multiple sclerosis, there is a very high probability that the other twin is likewise affected: one in three.[xii]

FAMILIES WITH SCLEROSIS

For cousins and other relatives, there is a low shared risk. About 80% of sclerosis patients know of no family members affected.[119,205]

The controversy about environment and genetics is still heated. What seems most likely is that the cause of multiple sclerosis is multifactorial —that is, involving several factors, both genetic and environmental ones, which coincide in the person who actually develops the disease. But in the "blood relative" forms of multiple sclerosis, genetics clearly matter more than the environment: siblings are affected to the same extent even when they live in different regions or climates.[5]

THE HEIRS GET ILL SOONER

As with other diseases, the forms of multiple sclerosis with a stronger hereditary base also present an earlier onset of the symptoms.

The chances of a blood relative being afflicted with multiple sclerosis vary according to the age at which the first symptoms appear. The maximum risk is found in patients under 20 (8.9%) and the minimum after age 40 (1.3 %).[xiii]

SHOULD WE MRI THE FAMILY?

A tough question, with its ethical complications and economic repercussions: should we subject the siblings or descendants of MS patients to magnetic resonance imaging in order to look for evidence of the disease in their systems? Hyperintense lesions have been found in some family members who had experienced no symptoms of demyelination.[306]

4. Multiple sclerosis is environmental

We have seen that genetics are important in developing multiple sclerosis, but they are not alone: something in the environment must trigger the disease.

There are many people who are hereditarily "predisposed" but never suffer from MS. Others, from the same gene pool, do come down with the disease because at some point in time something happened in their immediate surroundings. We don't know if that "something" is a virus, a toxin, the climate, a special diet, or something else. We only know that the "contact" took place in childhood or adolescence, and that the symptoms appeared five, ten or twenty years later.

STAY CLOSE TO THE EQUATOR

The risk of being afflicted with multiple sclerosis varies with the geographical latitute: there is more likelihood of the disease among persons who live far from the equator (especially during their childhood-adolescence). In tropical regions, multiple sclerosis is hardly mentioned. Per 100,000 inhabitants in Florida there are 15 MS patients; but this figure increases to 80 in Boston, and over 100 in Scandinavia or Iceland.[84]

In our hemisphere, the farther north you go, the more cases you encounter, and the more serious the cases. For each patient who dies in New Orleans (30°N), five die in Boston (42°N).

If an American moves to the north of the country, his chances of suffering from multiple sclerosis increase.[270] The same is true in Japan, although the Japanese are less vulnerable to the disease.

In the southern hemisphere, the disease also predominates in the zones farthest from the equator, this time to the south.[334]

THE RACE OF PHAËTON

In Ethiopia, Libya and other sunny desert lands there is no multiple sclerosis. According to mythology, the deserts were formed after the wild race of Phaëton, son of Helios, who convinced his father to let him take the carriage of the Sun out for a drive one day.

The spirited steeds who moved the great ball of fire around the Earth (Greek mythology is pre-Copernican) ran out of control and got too close to our planet's surface at some spots, charring it, leaving arid desert regions.

The geographical areas that Phaëton[xiv] approached in his race have no multiple sclerosis patients. The desert and the sun protect them, it seems. Ethiopians (*"burned faces"* in Greek[20]) are not affected by the disease.

The climate and the amount of solar radiation influence the appearance of multiple sclerosis,[277] which prefers cold, rainy regions.[288]

WORLD WAR II INVADERS

He was an English soldier who had just turned 20 before arriving on the island.

He did not know that half a century later he would be accused of introducing a terrible disease there. He belonged to a British battalion (the year is 1940) with orders to occupy the Faeroe Islands[xv] islands before Hitler´s boats could.

These islands had never had a case of multiple sclerosis. After the occupation (1943-1960) though, 24 cases were reported, a real epidemic for such a small population.[272] And later, virtually nothing: just one patient in thirty years. Something similar happened in Iceland.[271]

RUSSIAN CHILDREN WHO EAT MEAT

Russian children who eat lots of meat run a greater risk of suffering from multiple sclerosis. The same observation has been made among children who have repeatedly suffered from amygdalitis (swollen tonsils) or from allergies before the age of 15.[196]

It is not the meat in itself; what increases the risk of the disease is the custom of smoking the meat, say researchers from France, Switzerland and the Faeroe Islands.[282,283]

In Croatia, multiple sclerosis has been associated not only with smoked meats, but also with a greater intake of animal fats, potatoes and unpasteurized milk.[485] Note, however, that we are talking here about statistical probabilities whose clinical significance is relative.

NO MORE MERCURY FILLINGS

The mouths of many people still have amalgam fillings that may contain mercury. It was a resistant and inexpensive means of restoring teeth decayed by time and caries. They were not very esthetically pleasing fillings, however, and they are no longer used. Dentists now have modern materials that are prettier and more costly. And, though it has not been conclusively shown, the new materials are beyond the suspicions raised around mercury amalgams.[xvi] The hypothesis is that, over time, the body absorbs the metal, which is toxic for the organism in general, and also increases the risk of developing multiple sclerosis.[489]

POLLUTION

Areas that are heavily contaminated have a negative influence on a person's health, and modify the body's defenses. This is the factor pointed out by some to support their studies that find more multiple sclerosis in polluted industrial zones, especially those related with the textile industry and metal processing (in France and the Czech Republic). The exogenous adverse components presumably lead to an important alteration of the immunological mechanisms, and have a triggering effect in multiple sclerosis.[358,284,295]

LIGHT, MORE LIGHT!

Licht, mehr licht![xvii] These were the famous last words of Goethe. The desire for light must be shared by persons susceptible to myelin problems, because sunlight protects us from multiple sclerosis.[226] Solar radiation and other climactic factors may determine whether or not the disease appears.[277] Countries with more hours of daylight have fewer patients, perhaps because the light or the ultraviolet rays have an immunosuppressive effect on the pineal gland.[226,335,383]

The pineal gland produces melatonin, the rhythm hormone, which also modulates immunity. With age, its importance diminishes, and 40% of normal adults have a calcified pineal gland. In multiple sclerosis, the calcification of the gland is premature and more intense. In one study it was found that all the MS patients had a calcified pineal gland;[467] these researchers deduced that certain anomalies of the pineal gland and the body's melatonin favor the development of the disease.

THE WELL MYELINATED POOR

The poor have better myelin than the rich. There is more multiple sclerosis among the well-educated and well-to-do.[42] Recent data[274] are conclusive: the disease is more frequent in people from the upper socioeconomic level. This can be seen even more clearly in developing countries, where differences in economic status and sanitary conditions are greater.[564]

Wealth affords no protection against multiple sclerosis.

AFRAID OF CHICKENPOX

Where varicella abounds, multiple sclerosis abounds. And vice versa. It is not unusual for the varicella or "chickenpox" virus (herpes zoster) to be involved in the pathogeny of multiple sclerosis. In high risk zones, this virus affects children before they reach age 10 (in 95% of children) and may be "dormant" (in a latent state) for many years, with periodic exacerbations as seen in multiple sclerosis.

One of those adhering to this hypothesis is Dr. Ross. With the excessive enthusiasm that characterizes new converts, he waged a campaign on the radio and in the papers announcing all over the U.S that varicella produces multiple sclerosis. That was in 1995. Millions of Americans were frightened by a theory that is still unfounded.

THE LAGGING VIRUS AND THE LATE VACCINE

The typical childhood illnesses should come along "on time"; that is, during childhood. Likewise, the vaccines should be given as scheduled by the pediatrician. Or else, problems may arise.

In one group of patients with multiple sclerosis, it was discovered that they had been vaccinated against polio at a late age, after their fifteenth birthdays.[49] Other studies found that the "common" childhood infections (measles, chickenpox, whooping cough and others) had affected the patients later than usual (statistically speaking).[320,38] Some of the females had had an early menarch (first menstrual period), which meant an increased risk of having "childhood illnesses" after reaching puberty.[380]

AN INFECTION SETS OFF THE MS

Multiple sclerosis is an immunological disease, with a genetic **and/or**[xviii] environmental basis, probably triggered by a virus.[94,242] We do not know which virus[xix] (in the form of an infection or a vaccine?) might have interacted with the patient during the early part of his life, favoring the appearance of the disease in adulthood. It may not be one germ alone: maybe this autoimmune disease is the "final junction" of several infections common to childhood that appeared in a specific order or intensity in a predisposed child.[86]

THE MYSTERIOUS DEATH OF MY CAT

"When I was a kid, I loved to play with my cat. But one day he got sick and died suddenly, we never knew what from." Tales like this were told quite frequently in the MS patient surveys done in Ohio.[221]

Among these patients, it was surprisingly common to have lost a cat to an unidentified disease during childhood or adolescence. Other studies have fine-tuned the theory to find more multiple sclerosis among former owners of siamese cats in particular.[209] If we accept the premise that a virus plays a role in multiple sclerosis, it is feasible that the infection could originate in humans or in animals.

DOGS WITH DISTEMPER

Other animals have had to shoulder the blame, too. Dogs, for instance. Puppies, if not vaccinated properly, run a high risk of contracting canine distemper. It is a disease produced by a neurotropic[i] virus which —apparently— does not harm man, though theoretically the virus might be transmitted to man.

No one has been able to demonstrate that multiple sclerosis is facilitated by the transmission of the distemper virus to man, but this controversial hypothesis would fit into the chronological scheme of increased incidence of MS in the Faeroe Islands, Iceland and other places.[89,92,93,95,424] Some recent studies insist on the role of the canine distemper virus.[94,345,346,439]

THE MYSTERY OF THE VILLAGE OF HENRIBOURG

Only 70 people live in this small Canadian village. One woman resident, back in the 40´s, was diagnosed with multiple sclerosis. She provided information that led doctors to discover that the disease coincided in six of her former classmates, as well as two soldiers who had been stationed in the area around the same time.[198]

Too many coincidences. Something was the matter in Henribourg, Saskatchewan. According to the Encyclopedia Britannica,[xx] this naturally beautiful Canadian province is the main region of passage for numerous songbirds, aquatic birds, falcons and owls, many of which make their nests there...

A BIRD ON THE WIRE, THEN IN THE POT[xxi]

Birds (except the two in the bush) may be vectors in the multiple sclerosis puzzle. They are believed to transmit the Epstein-Barr virus, and antibodies to this virus tend to be plentiful in multiple sclerosis patients.[307,333,366,541]

Others say that the disease strikes persons who eat stew made with seagulls infected with ornithosis.

During Wold War II the inhabitants of the Faeroe Islands stewed and ate some types of aquatic birds.[282] So it may be, after all, that the British invasion is not to blame for the infamous epidemic of sclerosis at that time in history.

GETTING OVERLY DEFENSIVE

Immunological hyperactivity: defense reactions are excessive and out of control in patients with multiple sclerosis. Their immune systems overrespond or respond improperly to a virus or other foreign element. This is the standing conclusion after determining that multiple sclerosis patients produce an excess of antibodies not just to one but to a number of viruses.[498] This can be seen in the blood, but better yet when the cerebrospinal fluid (CSF) is analyzed. It's not a matter of reacting to a latent virus, then, but rather that these patients misreact to a great variety of viral agents.

A SYSTEMIC DISEASE

In multiple sclerosis, the genetic characteristic that is transmitted is a systemic condition, which is asymptomatic at first, and not restricted to the nervous system; other alterations can be seen, for example, in the leukocytes.[123] Later on, the environment would be determinant in the evolution of the inherited genetic trait. This would explain the low concordance of the disease in monozygotic twins.[410]

MORE AND MORE MS

As ever-changing as a weathervane, multiple sclerosis is instable even with regard to its frequency. In a single country the incidence varies over the years or even over shorter time periods. In Norway[337] there was a noteworthy increase from 1975 to 1985. In the Shetland Islands[93] incidence is on the decline, with a major drop documented for the period 1951-1968.

Returning to Norway, periodic fluctuations have been described.[121] Others say that the variations in incidence come at the expense of a certain specific evolutive form, meaning that there are several types of multiple sclerosis.[280] From a historical standpoint, most data point to a slight increase in the extension of the disease.[71,121,330,473,546]

VITAMIN D ON TRIAL

Epidemiological studies show one strange coincidence: in the places where there is more multiple sclerosis, there are also more cases of prostate cancer, dental caries, colon cancer, and Parkinson's disease. Some even dare to offer an explanation: these clinically diverse diseases may share an aberration to vitamin (hormone) D, which plays a multifarious role in immunoregulation.[478]

CIRCUMSTANTIAL EVIDENCE?

Among women with multiple sclerosis there are many hairdressers[500] and nurses.[209] Among men, there are more who work with metal, or in electric companies.[287] For both men and women, visiting military bases is more common.[209] and blood type O positive stands out.[318,323]

Is the connection one of chance or necessity?[xxii]

CLASSICAL HYPOTHESES

Intuition is a shortcut to knowledge. I like to heed the words, even when unaccompanied by proof, of intelligent people, be they neurologists or poets. Shakespeare's tragedies offer the outlines of modern psychoanalysis. Simple observations made by Charcot or Parkinson contain brilliant ideas that were to become banners for scientists many years later. Medical hypotheses must be tested in controlled studies, but proposing them in the theoretical realm is an exercise in imagination and intelligence that can open doors to future solutions. Or, the notions may live on as simple anecdotes.

The great figures of medicine at the beginning of this century offered a long list of factors they believed to be related with multiple sclerosis: sweat,[98] stress,[76,165] exposure to the cold, excessive effort, previous acute infections (typhoid fever, smallpox) a circulating myelinolytic toxin (literally, one that "breaks up" the myelin),[315] etc.

AS CAREFREE AS THE WIND

They are modern fancies, hypotheses uttered carelessly, in the absence of demonstrations or rigorous methodology. But they just might contain a grain of truth about the causes and mechanisms behind multiple sclerosis.

- Abuse of medication and other drugs.[61]

- Alterations in the oligodendrocytes: due to the incapacity of the precursor cells,[122] to a viral infection,[308] or to an attack by prions.[xxiii] (556)

- The responsibility for the demyelination lies with the astrocytes, those helpful executive cells that contribute to the processes of healing and regeneration.[214]

- The initial nerve lesion has a vascular origin: there are genetically susceptible vessels that produce local hypertension (high blood pressure), and ischemic hypoxia. This sets off the demylinating process and the secondary disturbances that alter the immunological system.[184] Along the same lines, but before birth: vascular and inflammatory alterations of the chorionic villi (of the placenta) take place in the mother of those who later suffer from multiple sclerosis and other autoimmune diseases.[276]

- The cause lies in the neurovegetative system. This theory is supported by the observation that the symptoms change according to changes in temperature, and that one out of every three women affected stops having a menstrual period.[254]

- Substance P plays a part in the formation of plaques. Substance P is a peptide neurotransmitter composed of eleven amino acid residues that regulates the immune response.[26]

- A virus is quartered in the sensory spinal ganglia and the craniospinal ganglia. Later, from these "privileged sanctuaries," it periodically invades the brain, the spinal cord or even (in other demyelinating diseases) the peripheral nerves.[368]

SOMETHING HAPPENED BEFORE AGE 15

Studying emigrants (or immigrants, depending on your point of view), we obtain clues as to whether the cause of a disease is genetic or environmental, though there may be a series of methodological difficulties involved.[168]

Sweden has a lot of multiple sclerosis, Ethiopia none. If a Swede were to move to Ethiopia and come down with multiple sclerosis, it would be because it was in his genetic makeup. If an Ethiopian emigrated to Sweden and were afflicted, it would be because something in the Nordic atmosphere facilitated the disease.

By studying migrant populations, we arrive at the conclusion that what matters is the age when one moved.

If an Ethiopian older than 15 years of age settles in Sweden, he will never have multiple sclerosis, but if he moves there during infancy he might (though he is still at less risk than the native Swede). Studies of emigrants support the importance of the environmental factor when there is a long incubation period.[102,168,268]

GENETICS TANGLED UP IN THE ENVIRONMENT

Genetics is very important, granted. But those contracting the disease must have been in contact with some environmental factor before reaching adulthood. Something happens before age 15 to precipitate, in genetically predisposed persons, the development of multiple sclerosis. Whatever one's ethnic background, an individual who moves to another country as an infant will take on the odds of the area he moved to. If he moves after adolescence, he goes with the odds of the country where he spent his childhood.[290]

Solid data are now available about the genetic bases of the disease and the necessity of a contributing environmental factor.[118,413,458,460,520] With the knowledge we possess today, it seems clear that the coincidence of both factors produces an autoimmune disorder in the patient. Genetics and the environment, all tangled up like blackberry branches on a fence.[xxiv]

5. The main symptoms

Multiple sclerosis can produce almost any symptom. The lesions, be they few or many, attack some part of the nervous system at random. Double or blurred vision, a staggering gait, arms that tingle or legs that feel like cardboard are the most frequent complaints. Also, trouble urinating or with bowel movements, problems with sexual activity, or changes in mood. Anything is possible.

The way in which these symptoms become manifest (their clinical evolution) is unpredictable. Most often, they appear in the form of "attacks" (exacerbations) that are repeated later (recurrent), alternating with periods of improvement. Other times the disturbances progress slowly and insidiously.

DISPERSE IN TIME AND IN SPACE

Dispersion is what characterizes the symptoms. They are disperse over time –some symptoms appear earlier, others later, with months or years of difference. And they are disperse spatially in the nervous system: damage to the cerebellum causes tremor, lesion of the sensitive fibers produces tingling, vision is impaired because there is a plaque in the brain stem, and legs are immobilized because the pyramidal tract is affected.

Multiple sclerosis is the epitome of a disperse disease.

THE STEALTHY ARRIVAL

Its rare for a patient to come to the neurologist with the first flare-up. At first, two or more mild symptoms usually coincide for a brief time, and they are subjective (the patient notices them but others "can't tell").

About half of the patients begin with tingling sensations or fatigue in one extremity, and one out of four with visual impairment. What makes them go to the doctor are the more pronounced symptoms (which are less frequent at the onset) such as paralysis, blindness, or important problems with balance.

AVANT-LA-LETTRE SYMPTOMS

They are the "in advance" symptoms (*avant-la-lettre*),[i] the ones that occurred before diagnosis. The patient may not have paid them much notice, or forgot them, but the doctor will insist on recollection in order to determine when the disease really began. Those problems with one leg that the patient thought was "sciatica"; the days when he or she saw double, "until glasses solved the problem"; or that period of dizzy spells after "a bout of the flu."

MINUTES, HOURS, DAYS, WEEKS OR MONTHS

How long does it take for the disturbances to become apparent? In this sense, too, everything about multiple sclerosis is variable, but the **rule of five** can serve as a guideline: out of every five patients, one will develop the symptoms in a matter of minutes (superacute forms), one in hours (subacute), one in a few days (acute), one over weeks (subchronic) and the other spaced out over months (chronic forms, more frequent after age 45).[3]

THE MOST FREQUENT SYMPTOMS

When the disease is established, the most frequent symptom (in nearly half of patients) is muscular weakness. It may be a feeling of "general" fatigue, or the complete paralysis of a specific area. The next most common is optic neuritis, in four out of every ten patients. One third has sensitive disturbances (ranging from abnormal sensations to real anesthesia). One fourth of our patients will show cerebellar tremor or problems with coordination. Following, in order of frequency, are nystagmus, diplopia (double vision) and incontinence.

THE FATIGUE THAT NO ONE SEES

Fatigue is the symptom that multiple sclerosis sufferers complain of most.[534] They are tired, exhausted even, and no one pays any attention. Since there is no paralysis, the family members do not acknowledge the problem (*"Oh, you're always saying you're so tired when nothing is wrong with you!"*) and even the doctor may not realize it (fatigue is not an objective sign —it cannot be measured). In fact, even the patient is sometimes not able to find words to describe the strange way he or she feels.

MIDBRAIN AND FATIGUE

The ascending reticular substance is a neuronal complex involved in wakefulness and keeping us active. It is situated in the brain stem, predominantly in the higher portions (midbrain or mesencephalon). It is precisely there where more demyelinating lesions can be seen when patients who suffer most from fatigue undergo magnetic resonance imaging.[108,349]

SPINAL CORD AND PARALYSIS

The muscular weakness may be intense and produce true paralysis of one or more extremities. It is a spastic paralysis; that is, there is an increased muscle tone and exaggeration of the tendinous reflexes. It happens because there are plaques in the spinal cord, more specifically, in the pyramidal motor tract, which carries the brain's orders to execute voluntary movements. In these patients, Babinski´s sign appears: when the bottom of the foot is scratched, the toes do not turn downward, as in a normal subject. Instead, they extend and fan out, especially the big toe.

THE SPINAL MEDULLA AND ATAXIA

If the plaques affect the medulla in the posterior funiculi, the cords that transmit deep sensitivity, the individual is capable of feeling pain and certain types of touch, but does not receive adequate information about the position of his limbs and the ground beneath him.

Then, upon walking, he lacks feedback about how he is moving, and his gait becomes incoordinated, ataxic. He staggers as if drunken. The lack of information from the feet and hands must be compensated by sight, by looking down continuously while walking. When the neurologist examines the patient, he makes him stand and close his eyes; and the patient, with no information to guide him, falls. This is known as the Romberg test.

LOST AND FOUND EYESIGHT

Suddenly, in a matter of hours or days, vision in one eye is lost, and the opthalmologist diagnoses optic neuritis. Of these cases, 90% recover sight spontaneously, but it may mark the onset of multiple sclerosis. Not all cases of optic neuritis evolve into multiple sclerosis, but there is a close relationship between the two. The attacks of optic neuritis are repeated in one out of four patients.

CEREBELLUM AND COORDINATION

The cerebellum is an organ specialized in integrating and coordinating movements. When plaques affect it, the symptoms appearing are dysmetria, dysarthria, dysdiadochokinesia, ataxic gait and intention tremor. This affection has a poor prognosis, especially when it appears in the initial stages of multiple sclerosis.

BRAIN STEM AND PAIRED CRANIAL NERVES

In the brain stem, besides the ascending and descending tracts, are the nuclei of the paired cranial nerves. When affected, damage may be done to the nerves responsible for sensitivity or movement of the face (trigeminal neuralgia, facial paralysis), the nerves of the inner ear and equilibrium (hearing disturbances or vertigo), or those that move the eyes, the oculomotor nerves (the patient sees double or has a special tremor in his look called nystagmus) Nystagmus is an important sign, as it appears in more than half of the patients with chronic multiple sclerosis. It was described way back when by Charcot, in his classic triad.

DIPLOPIA OF THE FASCICULUS

When we look to the left, our left eye must move outward, and the right eye inward, and they must do this at the same time, coordinated. That is what the medial longitudinal fasciculus, which is a double nerve pathway. It connects the inner right ocular motor nucleus (which moves the right eye inward) with the left outer ocular motor nucleus (which moves the left eye outward), or vice versa.

If the fasciculus that serves to look to the left is damaged, the patient will see double when he tries to look in that direction, because the oculomotor nuclei are not coordinated (although they can move separately). This is what is known as opthalmoplegia internuclearis: the patient sees double when he looks to one side, but not to the other, or when the eyes converge to read. The lesion may be due to a sclerosis plaque or other causes (vascular, tumoral, etc.).[ii]

WHEN THERE IS NO CAPTAIN, THE SAILOR COMMANDS

If the brain cannot send orders to the spinal cord, then the latter does it on its own. The neurons in the medulla have their own circuits that allow it to react in an autonomous way to a stimulus. If a person steps on a sharp object, the medulla responds by retracting the foot (contracting the leg flexors) and it does it automatically, before the brain even "figures out" what is going on.

If a muscle in the thigh is stretched brusquely, there is also a circuit in the medulla that stops the action, making the muscle contract. This is the so-called stretch reflex,[ii] the one the neurologist provokes by tapping the tendon of the knee with his rubber hammer.[iii]

When plaques affect the pyramidal tract or other descending tracts, they are left without voluntary movement (there is paralysis), and in addition the medullar reflexes become independent, with no "captain" sending them orders. As a result, they exaggerate their activity, and contract the muscles too much, even when the stimuli are minimal. Hyperreflexia appears (reflexes are exaggerated) and spasticity is present (the increased tone of the muscles causes intense contractures). The patient remains immobile, with fixed positions that do not even yield to our attempts to move him passively.

TERMS OF SPASTICITY

At times spasticity is not continuous, but appears in the form of a crisis, or muscular spasms. They are episodes of variable duration in which one muscle or group of muscles are contracted, a sort of "cramp" or "charley horse" that is usually painful and occurs at night, and affects the lower extremities more often.

WOMEN FEEL THE PAIN MORE

Multiple sclerosis patients suffer considerably from their pains, sometimes from the very start of the disease. In fact, the form of presentation of the disease may be a chronic pain of unknown origen.[407] The pains are more intense and frequent among women (affected two or three times as often as men)[360,540] and in spastic forms of the disease. The acute pain presents itself as neuralgias, painful optic neuritis, or as Lhermitte´s sign. Chronic pain (lumbago, spasms, dysesthesias) is characteristic of medullary lesions.[360,503] Occasionally multiple sclerosis presents itself as an intense "headache" in a person with no history of migraines.[164]

THE MEDULLA IS HARD ON THE BLADDER

Bladder trouble arises when the plaques affect certain zones of the spinal cord.[159] The patients urinate more frequently (polaquiuria) and when they urininate, patients feel as if they had not finished (urinary tenesmus). At times the need to urinate is urgent or there is incontinence (leakage). Less frequent are problems of retention (the bladder cannot empty completely). In men, these symptoms are generally accompanied by impotence.

COMBINED FORMS

Half of multiple sclerosis patients have mixed or generalized clinical forms. The entire central nervous system appears affected to a greater or lesser degree, with a mixture of symptoms: medullary, cerebral, of the optic nerves, the cerebellum and brain stem. One third of patients present preferentially medullar forms, with spastic paralysis and ataxia. Only 5% have forms in which cerebellar symptoms or visual deficits are predominant (an optic neuritis that leaves sequelae).[3]

THE GRAY MATTER HAS BULL[iv]

Multiple sclerosis affects any part of the nervous system, but the gray matter —in cerebral cortex and basal ganglia— is almost never harmed.[3,441] That is why we rarely see symptoms like dementia, aphasia (difficulty putting thoughts into words), convulsions, coma, parkinsonism or other abnormal movements of the extrapyramidal sort.

6. Mind, mood and personality

Many doctors believe that multiple sclerosis produces no mental disturbances, or that these appear only in serious cases with a long evolution.[33] In fact, the routine neurological examination only discovers cognitive alterations in five percent of patients.[246,269,332]

Nonetheless, the mind, moods and personality are altered in most patients.[i] The causes are both primary (due to neurological damage) and secondary (because of stress and the mode of coping with a chronic disease) Sometimes these problems are more incapacitating than the physical sequelae.

STUPID INDIFFERENCE

Some multiple sclerosis patients give the impression that they could not care less about their disease. Charcot called this "stupid indifference," and Vulpian spoke of "morbid optimism" in describing their overly positive outlook.

They exhibit **euphoria**, a carefree or even jubilant state that is actually pathological. It is an inappropriate manner of reacting to the problems that plague them. The euphoria indicates that there are lesions in the white matter of the frontal lobes, and it is always accompanied by signs of cerebral affection.[3,161]

DETERIORATION FROM THE START

The tests we use to measure the dementia caused by Alzheimer's disease are of no use in multiple sclerosis patients, because most of them maintain language and intelligence in general.[428] But special testing reveals that half the patients suffer a slight cognitive deterioration from the very beginning of the disease,[64,259,406,427] which is more pronounced in the days following a flare-up.[156]

Over the years, visuo-spatial capacity, reckoning, recent memory, attention, information processing (verbal) and abstraction or the formation of concepts are all affected.[310] After three years, one in five patients shows considerable mental deterioration,[12,48,232,239,428] and these are the most incapacitated patients.[81]

THE DISCONNECTED CORTEX

The cognitive alterations are produced because the lesions of the white matter "disconnect" the cerebral cortex, isolating it.[418] Magnetic resonance imaging shows lesions around the ventricles, many of them coalescing, especially in the corpus callosum. Single photon emission computed tomography (SPECT) reveals defects in the frontal lobes.[416,417,419] The third ventricle may appear dilated and there may be cortical atrophy to some degree.[425]

BIOGRAPHICAL GAPS

When our memory fails, it is usually with regard to recent things ("Where did I leave that pen?"), but we remember early events from years back (schoolmates, summer camp).

In multiple sclerosis, it is the other way around: most patients maintain immediate or recent memory, but fail inexplicably when trying to recall important events of their childhood or adolescence. Family members are surprised by these biographical lapses, which are more frequent in the chronic-progressive forms of MS.[33-35,81]

STEADFAST IN THEIR ERRORS

They are not good at problem-solving because they insist on their misunderstandings and errors.

The multiple sclerosis patient gives "perseverant responses" in neuropsychological tests: he is unable to discard an incorrect or irrelevant hypothesis that others would give up on quickly.[34,207,429,430] This behavior takes hold when the plaques disconnect some of the circuits of the frontal lobes (it is also seen in traumatisms or tumors of this region of the brain).

LACONIC, BUT NOT FROM SPARTA

When someone speaks little, we say they are laconic, which is actually the same as calling them Spartan.[ii] Verbal fluency is diminished in these patients [34,66] for several reasons. They retrieve stored information slowly, which makes it difficult for them to "find the words." They may have dysarthria (difficulty in uttering sounds), and psychological problems are present as well.

Verbal fluency is worse if there are plaques in the anterior portion of the corpus callosum, in the frontal regions and in the left hemisphere.[416,419] Yet other types of problems with language, such as aphasia, alexia or agraphia, are rare.

THAT UNFAMILIAR FACE

Some patients have trouble recognizing familiar persons, or distinguishing the emotions reflected in a face.[430] The technical term for this is **prosopagnosia** (from *prosopos* = face or person, and *agnosia* = lack of knowledge) and it is characteristic of lesions in the right half of the brain (posterior section) which disrupt visual perception or the mode of processing visuo-spatial information.

LAUGHTER FROM A SIMPLE SOURCE

On occasions, they laugh or cry for no good reason. This pathological laughing and crying indicates an emotional lability[149] that we see in one out of every ten patients.

It is not related with the exacerbations, or with depression or anxiety. However, in the patients with "pathological laughter," there is intellectual imparirment.[134] Cervantes[74] did not need any statistical studies to come to the same conclusion in *Don Quixote*: "Laughter brought on by a slight cause is the sign of a simple mind."

DEMENTIA IS RARE

In some patients with a highly incapacitating long-term evolution of the disease, the mental deficit can be very intense, constituting real dementia,[iii] but fortunately, this is rare in multiple sclerosis.

In these rare cases, the dementia is "subcortical,"[484] of a "white matter" nature (affecting attention and psychomotor functions to a greater extent), unlike the Alzheimer type of dementia (with more verbal and memory impairment), which is of a "gray matter" nature.[148]

MENTAL ILLNESSES ARE CEREBRAL DISEASES

This old saying holds true for multiple sclerosis: mental or cognitive alterations (and, to some extent, affective and personality changes) reflect lesions produced in the brain. The more the plaques, the greater the damage and mental disturbance.

An analysis of magnetic resonance images points to a commonsense conclusion: patients with a greater total of hyperintense lesions also have a greater cognitive deficit,[349,444] especially when the lesions predominate in posterior periventricular regions and tend to coalesce.[176] Lesions in the temporal lobe produce more psychiatric disorders.[220]

HALF ARE DEPRESSED

Multiple sclerosis patients have an increased tendency to suffer from depression[iv] with respect to other groups of chronically ill persons[477]. According to different studies, depression affects between one-fourth[349] and one-half[376] of them.

The depression bears a close relation with the state of activity of the disease at that moment.[376] It is not related with age, sex, duration of the disease, cognitive deficit, incapacity, nor the type of lesions seen with magnetic resonance imaging.[349]

WOMEN AND PSYCHIATRY

Some 90% of the patients suffer from anxiety,[376] moreso when the sclerosis is in an active phase. If depression can be said to affect approximately 40% of patients, more than 10% meet criteria for bipolar (manic-depressive) disorder.[240] And they do not fit the "familiar" model for affective disorders.[241]

An association has been established between multiple sclerosis and affective disorders, in the patient and family members, which is more evident among women: of 31 patients with serious affective disorders, 27 were women.[475]

STAY AWAY FROM STRESS

We already know that stress[v] aggravates high blood pressure, cardiac disease, epilepsy and even cancer. And multiple sclerosis, too. Charcot said so a century ago, and now we have proof that he was right.

Stress has an influence on the appearance of flare-ups[vi] and might even be a conditioning factor in the development of the disease itself.[188,189,190,253, 507,542,543] A patient exposed to stressful situations or continuous stress is at a higher risk of suffering a relapse, and will have a worse long-term evolution of the disease.

This is logical: stress affects the immunological system,[77] which is already altered in multiple sclerosis.[vii]

THE SUICIDES CLUB

It is the title of a story by Robert Louis Stevenson.[506] ¿???? We can use it to emphasize —with literary exaggeration— the incresased risk of suicide among patients with multiple sclerosis. There are twice as many suicides among MS patients as compared with healthy persons.

A suicidal person may initially find himself or herself in situations of depression, which are frequent in multiple sclerosis. There are other contributing factors: stress at home, financial problems, social isolation, changes for the worse in one's lifestyle, and, above all, a lack of confidence in one's future (the latter would appear to be the most decisive factor, more than depression).[278]

The risk of suicide demands that depression be treated. Besides antidepressants, psychotherapy should be prescribed. Emphasis should be placed on available means of improving the quality of life, and on formulating realistic expectations, present and future, for new treatments. Autopsies have shown that the cerebra of suicide victims have low levels of serotonin (a precursor of melatonin), and that the pineal gland is low in melatonin. But we need to know this well ahead of time. A blood sample could be taken while the patient sleeps; if the melatonin levels are low, there may be a danger of suicide, calling for preventive measures.[469]

MS PERSONALITY

The personality of patients with multiple sclerosis might be influenced by genetics,[viii] or be a consequence of the social environment (family, education), or else a manner of reacting to the disease. Or maybe all of the above.

Patients themselves acknowledge their lack of emotional control and the tendency for the euphoria to increase over the years.[310] There is a characteristic mental profile of multiple sclerosis patients, in which affective disorders are associated with two specific trends: on the one hand, dysphoria, euphoria and mania; and on the other hand, depression, anxiety and a tendency to dramatize, with some degree of anosognosia (denial of the disease). This neuropsychological type is also seen in basal and medial lesions of the frontal lobes.[507]

The defense and coping mechanisms go through changes, and the psychiatrist must be on the alert.[376] These patients tend to resort to repression and self-isolation as compensating elements.[72]

WHAT THEY NEED IS LOVE

Multiple sclerosis patients have a special need for affection, but they request this love in a passive form.[107] Their self-esteem depends on the fulfillment of this need for affection in the home and social realm.[538]

In terms of psychodynamics, they have rigid defense mechanisms, and difficulties in resolving their intimate conflicts, through either sublimation or the internalization of new and satisfying emotional experiences.

Multiple sclerosis patients have suffered more than usual in childhood, with unpleasant events taking place at an early age. This, in some patients, conditions personality in an altered structure.[107]

They also have more traits associated with depression and self-aggression (after all, self-immunity is a sort of attack on oneself).

CHRONIC GRIEF

It is not true depression, but rather a melancholy vein detected in the personality of these patients. Most of them suffer from "chronic grief," a lasting sadness or downspirited tendency, that gets worse at certain times.[199,200,539]

DEPRESSION AND THE LIMBIC SYSTEM

The cause of the depression in these patients may be affectation of the limbic system. By studying the regional brain flow (by SPECT), asymmetries have been observed in the limbic system of depressed patients as compared with control subjects.[457] It has also been observed that the mood of MS patients is related to neuro-endocrinological disorders, due to affectation of the hypothalamus and hypophysis.[129]

DENTAL AND MENTAL HEALTH

Multiple sclerosis sufferers have normal dental health, but more problems with the temporomaxillary joint.[513] Among the group with greater pschiatric problems, there are also more dental fillings, in which mercury amalgams may have been used. The toxicity of mercury, some say, could cause multiple sclerosis. Though that hypothesis seems a bit far-fetched, some studies do show that the more the mercury, the more the mental disorders.[489]

A STRAITJACKET FOR SCLEROSIS

An MS patient who has no history of psychiatric problems may suddenly present signs of psychosis. This would be an exacerbation of the disease that has affected, principally or exclusively, the hemispheric white matter. The proof is in the resonance and the study of immunoglobulins in the cerebrospinal fluid (CSF).[78,135,215,225] Some "psychotic" patients, who may end up in a mental hospital (or similar), are patients with "encephalitic" variants of multiple sclerosis or of other neurological diseases. After all, *mental illnesses are cerebral diseases.*

PERSONALIZED HANDWRITING

Graphology is the study of handwriting as an indication of temperament or personality. Writing is a unique characteristic of human behavior, requiring the integration of numerous circuits: motor, sensory, of coordination and language. When a neurological disease damages these circuits, a disturbance in handwriting will result. Graphologists can analyze it using physical and psychological criteria.

There is one very specific graphological method useful in determining the typical alterations of multiple sclerosis.[547] The analyses of these graphological techniques are much more exact nowadays, thanks to the help provided by computer processing programs.

AS YOU ARE, SO YOU LOVE

Words of wisdom from Ortega y Gasset, a Spanish philosopher. Love is the most delicate and all-encompassing act of the mind.[ix] If disease damages the brain (the mind), it may alter a person's capacity for love and tenderness, the most elaborate affect display.

Affective disorders (dysphoria, depression and anxiety) in multiple sclerosis patients are going to modify their loving relationships, in one way or another. The personal traits of the spouse or companion, and their attitude toward the disease, are very important. In this sense, it has been shown that women are more helpful than men, both directly and indirectly, for example in securing necessary resources and facilitating social integration.[180]

SINGING WHAT IS LOST

So goes a verse sung by Amancio Prada[x] (but written by the great poet Antonio Machado[309]). The nostalgia we feel with regards to lost capacities affects all humans, and in chronically ill patients it can be a dangerous sentiment. Fortunately, adaptation is better over time. When something negative upsets our lives, we develop mechanisms for coping or overcoming. To paraphrase Sartre, we've got to do something with what life has done to us. Each individual responds differently to adversity, depending on their personal capacities and upbringing.

In association with multiple sclerosis, the most negative reactions are seen in young patients, and in those who have had the disease for just a few years. Later on, evolution is more positive: over time, the problem is accepted, mechanisms of compensation are developed, and there is a higher degree of satisfaction and social adaptation.[455] The patient has to stop looking at the past in order to face the future with realistic expectations.

7. Sex, sphincters and other symptoms

Sex, the motor of life, is especially important in young persons, such as those who develop multiple sclerosis. Some are able to continue their sexual relationships without any real problems; others are not. When difficulties do arise, they coincide with urinary problems or depression[25,325] and they increase as the years go by.[505] We shall have a look at them here, together with some other less frequent symptoms of multiple sclerosis.

FETISHISM

His coworkers considered him an ordinary young man until they found out that he collected women's underwear. The diagnosis was made by magnetic resonance imaging: there were demyelinating plaques in the temporal and the frontal lobes.[227] The malfunction had manifested itself as a fetish, a form of hypersexuality or sexual deviation, as described by Freud. In multiple sclerosis patients, however, hypersexuality is not common. Quite the contrary.

THE HEN THAT DOESN'T EAT HAS ALREADY EATEN

Her husband lost all interest in sex. He was not impotent; he simply never tried to touch her any more. The woman was young and attractive, and until then their sex life had been very satisfactory, so she talked it over with a close friend. The friend minced matters with a barnyard metaphor: "*The hen that doesn't eat has already eaten*; your husband is having an affair."

Neither of the two could imagine that the husband had multiple sclerosis. In 65% of these patients there is a decrease in sexual activity, sometimes occurring even before the diagnosis. Once they know, one out of every three patients loses interest in sex and lovemaking.[325]

ERECTION, LUBRICATION AND PLEASURE

Men suffer from more sexual dysfunctions. Out of three men with multiple sclerosis, two will have erections that are too short or weak to make penetration possible.

In women, the problem is with lubrication. There is difficulty in achieving orgasm, and both men and women enjoy sex less than they used to. The lack of orgasm is experienced more in patients with pyramidal symptoms and plaques in the brainstem.[25]

BLOWING UP BALLOONS

Blowing up an air balloon is not enough; you've got to make sure the air does not escape. In a normal erection, excitation makes the muscles in the arteries relax, and the penis fills with blood; but something has to trap the blood there.

There are devices that imitate this process. The flaccid penis is put in a vacuum tube where we create negative pressure (manually or automatically) which makes blood flow into the erectile tissue. To maintain the erection, a rubber band is placed around the base of the penis (for no more than 20 minutes).[155] Consultation with a doctor is an absolute must.

NATURAL AND ARTIFICIAL MASTURBATION

Some men cannot have an erection because of psychological problems. Others get sexually excited, but have lesions on the descending nerve pathways, and the "order" does not reach the sacral cord, which plays a key role in erection. If the medullar reaction of erection exists, we can provoke it locally instead of mentally, that is, stimulating the penis by natural masturbation (the patient himself or with the help of his sexual companion), or using a vibrator. If necessary, the rubber band might be used at the base of the penis to prolong the erection.

DINNER AND THEN "VIAGRA"

Viagra is the latest drug craze. It may improve erection considerably (ejaculation is not guaranteed), and it is so easy to use that some men have no second thoughts about its high price.

USA Today published the comments of a man in his fifties who had been resorting to bothersome penile injections for many years, and then tried the new miracle drug. His formula was simple: take the lady out to dinner, and pop a Viagra for dessert. Enthusiastic tales like this one helped the stock of the pharmaceutical laboratory go sky-high. However, a number of complications and risks associated with this treatment have also been reported recently. Talk it over with the doctor.

PSYCHIC, REFLEX OR CREAM LUBRICATION

When a woman is sexually aroused, her vagina becomes moist. This lubrication has a psychic origin, and it may fail in patients with multiple sclerosis, either due to a lack of libido or because the descending tracts are lesioned. In such a case, lubrication can be provoked as a reflex, as we described for men, through natural or artificial masturbation previous to intercourse. Lubricating creams would be another alternative.

A TOWEL BETWEEN THE LEGS

In women with spasticity of the adductor muscles, the thighs may be held firmly together, "closed," creating problems for intercourse. Penetration may be attempted from a lateral position. If this does not help enough, a towel can be placed between the woman's knees.[155]

SEX IS A VARIED PLATTER

Sex can be thought of as a game, and as such, governed by rules that are established through a code of conduct between consenting adults.[i] Patients should get to know their limitations and possibilities in the sexual domain, and, in agreement with their mate, obtain the gratification that the new situation permits.

The search for new postions for sexual intercourse enriches the relations of any couple. If one of them has problems due to spasticity or osteomuscular alterations, using some imagination in trying new positions can have a twofold positive effect, physical and psychic.

CORTICOIDS AS APHRODISIACS

Surprisingly, the corticoids most commonly used in treating other symptoms of multiple sclerosis (motor or sensitive disturbances, lack of coordination, etc.) have also been reported to improve sexual functions. For what reason, we do not really know.[325]

GOOD PREGNANCY AND BAD PUERPERIUM

The classic doctrine[ii] was that multiple sclerosis gets worse (or could even be brought on by) pregnancy. Until not long ago, pregnant MS patients were advised to abort. Now we know that exacerbations of multiple sclerosis are less frequent precisely during the months of gestation, above all in the last trimester,[263] which is when the levels of alpha-AFP (a powerful natural immunosuppressor) are highest.[253]

But the puerperium is risky indeed. One in three patients has a flare-up in the months right after giving birth. If we look at an entire year (the nine months of gestation and three of puerperium), the total risk of having a relapse is doubled.[486,338] And yet the number of relapses does not always mean greater incapacity, and some very long-term studies point to favorable effects associated with childbearing.[456] (See chapter 17 for more details.) The exacerbations increase in number in the first three months after giving birth, and are slightly more frequent (but not significantly so) among the mothers who breastfeed.[369]

PREGNANCY, SCLEROSIS AND ARTHRITIS

Gestation has an influence on the evolution of rheumatoid arthritis and multiple sclerosis, and the changes produced are similar. Both are autoimmune diseases, and correlating their modifcations during pregnancy might provide new etiopathogenic data.[101]

TROUBLE STORING URINE

The patient has to run to the toilet (urgency) or go very often (polaquiuria, not to be confused with poliuria[iii]). It is more common just after the onset of multiple sclerosis in patients with bilateral lesions of the pyramidal tract. The sphincter (the circular muscle that closes the bladder) is normal, but the musculature is irritable (spastic) and won't settle down. The problem is very bothersome, and may improve if the detrusor is relaxed with anticholinergic drugs: imipramine (Tofranil), oxybutinin (Ditropan) or propantheline. They may cause dryness of the mouth, tachycardia, or poor visual accomodation. A recent study advocates the use of capsaicin infusions for serious hyperreflexia of the detrusor.[552]

THE BLADDER DOES NOT EMPTY PROPERLY

This is seen in later stages. The reason is that the sphincter remains contracted (always closed), or the muscle of the bladder (detrusor) is weak and cannot "push" well, or both. The bladder is flaccid, it expands because it gets full and does not empty completely, and some urine remains after miction. This vesical residue must be avoided, because it facilitates chronic infections.

Massaging or pressing on the area, from up to down, can help empty a bladder that is paralyzed. But it should not be done if the detrusor won´t relax, because then the urine that cannot evacuate through the urethra will flow up into the kidneys and favor infections there. In patients with a flaccid bladder and large amounts of residual urine it is necessary to void with catheters several times a day. Unless the patient is highly incapacitated, it is preferable to train him (or her) to use the catheter alone, as independence is an important consideration.

THE BLADDER AND SPHINCTER ARE DIVORCED

The technical term is detrusor-sphincter dyssynergia. It is a special situation in which the bladder muscle and the sphincter that closes it cannot work together. The result is a mixed condition, with urgency in urinating or incontinence alternating with urinary retention. Many times treatment will involve both anticholinergic therapy and the intermittant use of a catheter. Prazosin can be used to decrease the dyssynergia between sphincter and detrusor because it relaxes the internal sphincter.

SECRET INCONTINENCE

Sometimes they won't tell the doctor. Or maybe they do, but the doctor doesn't think it is all that important. In either case, the patient is stuck with the problem of incontinence. An English physician, Dr. Isaacs, gets to the heart of the matter with this aphorism:

"Attitudes toward incontinence are a mixture of antipathy, apathy, sympathy and empathy. Antipathy is disgust, apathy is distance, sympathy is care, empathy is action. The antipathetic doctor scolds, the apathetic one probes, the sympathetc doctor looks sad and the empatheic doctor investigates and treats."

And most bladder problems should be treated, above all if the neurologist and urologist are in contact with each other.[113] The need for this interchange between specialists is evident if we look at the high frequency of vesicular problems among multiple sclerosis patients: in more than half the total number of patients, and an even higher percentage of those with secondary progressive forms or with important pyramidal and cerebellar affectation.[23,63] In incontinence and urgency, and particularly in men, rehabilitation exercises for the muscles of the perineum are effective, sometimes with the help of electrical stimulation.[530]

FECAL INCONTINENCE IS RARE

There may be some fecal incontinence in cases of multiple sclerosis patients, but it is rare and other possible causes must be looked into. In patients with weakness or anesthesia from the waist down, the rectal sphincter is relaxed and fecal incontinence may be a problem. Usually, over time the patient regains some control by learning to contract other muscles in the peroneum. Some antibiotics used for urinary infections produce diarrhea and make incontinence worse.

There is a need to develop the habit of defecating regularly, always after meals, reinforcing the gastrocolic reflex. In very rare instances a colostomy (surgical intervention to expel feces through a bag in the abdominal surface) is performed; it should never be done until a year has passed and all other measures have been tried.

LIGHTENING DOWN MY BACK

"I went to turn my head and suddenly I felt something like lightening, a sort of electrical current that ran down my back, to my legs, which tingled. This happened two or three more times when I bowed my head. Then it never came back."

The patient is describing Lhermitte's sign,[iv] very characteristic of multiple sclerosis (appearing in one out of three patients). But it is not pathognomic,[ii] as it is observed in other pathologies involving.the spinal cord, most often due to spondylosis or a traumatism that has left a small scar on the medullary meninges.[522] If this is an isolated sign in a young person, the possibility of multiple sclerosis can be excluded.

THE *CALDARIUM* TEST

Actually it is known as the hot bath test, but since that was a favorite Roman pasttime, I prefer to use their name for it: Caldarium.[v] It is an ill-advised practice for multiple sclerosis patients. If a patient takes a hot bath, his symptoms may come back or get worse (reported in 80% of the cases), or new ones might even appear (in 60%). The disturbances brought on by the hyperthermia tend to pass after two or three hours, and some patients even experience a rebound phase of "well-being."

The scientific explanation is basically that high temperatures slow down the conduction of the nerve impulses that were already slow because of the loss of myelin, although other factors are also involved (serum calcium levels, blockage of the ion channels, circulatory changes, proteins and other substances produced by the hyperthermia, etc.).[197]

BLINDED BY EXERCISE

In some patients, exercise provokes a transitory blindness (Uhthoff symptom[1]); this usually reveals an optic neuritis that was latent. The workings are similar to those of the hot bath test: certain metabolic by-products and an increase in temperature due to the physical effort cause a temporary blockage in the conduction of the demyelinated optic nerve.[483]

TYPICAL YET RARE

There are also some symptoms that are rarely observed in multiple sclerosis, yet when they do appear, they are very useful for diagnosis. Two we have seen already: Lhermitte´s sign and ophtalmoplegia internuclearis. Others are facial myokymia (spontaneous undulation of the facial muscles, not to be confused with benign tics); some painful tonic convulsions (from damage to the brainstem); and the appearance of trigeminal neuralgia in a young person (to be seen in the diagnosis).

"A BRAMBLE BUSH BETWEEN MY LEGS"[vi]

Others may say, *"It´s as if I had sand paper between my fingers,"* *"caterpillars in my stomach,"* or *"hot water flowing within me."* The abnormal sensations experienced may sound strange, and the weirdly imaginative descriptions may lead the patient to be considered hysterical.

These paresthesias (from *para* = abnormal, and *esthesia* = sensación). can occur in other neurological diseases, but in multiple sclerosis and hysteria they are particularly strange. They are more frequent than hypoesthesis or anesthesis (deficit or absence of sensation). Paresthesias take on many different expressions, and the patient often describes them in bizarre terms. Sometimes there is merely a sensation of pruritis (itching).[67]

Their location also varies: yesterday the patient felt them in her right leg, and today in her left arm, or in the genital area. In the days before magnetic resonance imaging there was no anatomical explanation for these strange paresthesias, which is why they were considered manifestations of hysteria.

LENDING A USELESS HAND

The patient moves his hand, but it is of no use, because he lacks articular sensitivity (he is not aware of the position of the fingers). The cause is a plaque on the posterior funiculi of the cervical medulla, which also decreases his fine sense of touch. Heat or pain are felt, and the strength and reflexes are normal. But his hand is "disconnected," and since he is not aware of its position, the patient stops using it.

PAROXYSMAL PHENOMENA

A previously healthy person starts to raise or twist her arm, or sometimes the leg of the same side, "as if dancing." Or else makes facial grimaces, overgesticulating. Normally they are treated with tranquilizers and then, several days later, these strange movements disappear. The family may well believe that the person was just nervous, or on the verge of hysteria.

Such is the presentation of choreas, spasms, dystonias and other abnormal movements that can affect an extremity, half of the face, or half of the body. They are paroxysmal phenomena (they appear without warning) or transitory abnormal movements (they last only days or weeks).[212] The most frequent causes are vascular problems or multiple sclerosis.[105,178,322,379,445] True epileptic crises are rare, and suggest that the plaques are near the cerebral cortex.[vii]

A DEVILISH COUGH

Another odd symptom is the one baptized *"diabolical cough"*, found in a non-smoking woman with multiple sclerosis who developed frequent crises of daytime or nighttime coughing, of a neurogenic nature and recurrent course, with no laryngeal or bronchial cause. Like most other paroxysmal phenomena, it went away after anti-epileptic treatment.[236]

THE PLAQUE THAT HELD UP THE PERIOD

It, too, is rare, but plaques may appear in the hypothalamus and produce endocrinal disturbances. One women aged 30 stopped menstruating (the condition is known as amenorrhea), and endocrinologists diagnosed her as lacking in gonadotrophic and somatotrophic hormones. Both of these are produced in the hypothalamus, where this patient had a plaque that was detected by magnetic resonance imaging.[100]

Other times subthalamic lesions have been seen to produce amenorrhea accompanied by galactorrhea (secretion of milk from the nipple).[516] Watch out, then, for the sudden appearance of endocrinological disturbances in association with multiple sclerosis.

THE BEATINGS OF A HEART AT SLEEP

In multiple sclerosis, the central lesions may alter the autonomous nervous system. Daily functional tests usually show normal, but studies carried out during sleep, or recording 24-hr periods, indicate a dysfunction of the sympathetic system, with a reduced adaptability to the variations of cardiac frequency.[37,173,350]

DREAMS IN OBLIVION

We always dream much more than we remember afterward. But in some nervous system disorders, above all those affecting the posterior regions of the brain, nearly all one's dreams are forgotton.

In patients with multiple sclerosis,[463] it is curious to note that during exacerbations they forget almost everything they dreamed. In addition, these patients have other problems at night: their sleep is fragmented, among other reasons because of painful nocturnal spasms, or periodical leg movements during sleep,[136] or due to the need to get up to urinate. Or, in some cases, as the result of small lesions in the brain stem.

SLEEPING BY DAY

They sleep poorly at night, and are drowsy during the day. In some cases, the excessive daytime drowsiness is a real problem. In fact, multiple sclerosis patients may suffer from narcolepsy (irresistible episodes of daytime sleep) or even cataplexy (sudden generalized muscle weakness, physiologically similar to that seen in REM sleep).[476]

Other sleep disorders have been described, such as the unusual type of sleep apnea known as "Ondine's curse."[viii] Plaques can be seen in the bulb (next to the area of reticular formation that controls automatic breathing). This can be quite dangerous, as there is a risk of sudden death.[21,179,396]

All these manifestations point to lesions in the areas of the brain stem that regulate sleep and involve serotonin, a neurotransmitter that is regulated by melatonin, which in turn is influenced by the pineal gland.[464] The mechanisms are complicated and not fully understood, but in patients with real narcolepsy or cataplexy, and even in those with daytime drowsiness, treatment with a new substance called modaphynyl proves effectivel.[54]

8. The diagnosis[i]

In diagnosing multiple sclerosis we will combine what the patient tells us, what the physician sees, and what tests reveal.

First the patient tells us about his subjective sensations (symptoms) and the order in which they appeared (clinical history or anamnesis) Then, the doctor, with the help of his hammer, needle or tuning fork, carries out a neurological examination in order to collect objective signs (Are the reflexes all right? Is there anesthesia? How is the patient´s gait?). Finally, complementary tests are called for: analytical, magnetic resonance, lumbar puncture, evoked potentials, and others.

UNITY IN DIVERSITY

The diagnosis is made when several symptoms --which are not in themselves specifically determinant-- form a fairly characteristic group. The presentation is more typical when the disease has advanced.

Over time, there are a succession of exacerbations and an accumulation of symptoms that can no longer be justified by one single lesion.

If an individual shows signs of muscular weakness, incoordination, defective vision, sensitive disturbances, and sexual or sphincter dysfunction, the doctor cannot attribute it to a tumor or a hemorrhage in some part of the body.

Such diverse symptoms are indicative of disperse lesions, and that is the main feature of multiple sclerosis.

DISPERSION IN TIME AND SPACE

Nowadays, the clinical diagnosis of multiple sclerosis is based on this double dispersion: temporal and spatial.

In time, because over months or years a number of episodes of neurological dysfunction have occurred. And in space, because the symptoms and signs indicate that there are several independent nervous lesions.

DIAGNOSING AT THE SECOND CHANCE

The first flare-up almost always goes unnoticed. Generally speaking, because the patient doesn't worry about the first symptoms (they are usually subjective: the patient complains but no one sees anything wrong), and besides, they tend to be slight and transitory.

In most cases, there is no diagnosis until the second exacerbation, and months or up to ten years may have gone by.[ii] In order to arrive at a diagnosis sooner, symptoms are not enough; complementary tests are needed. These most often include lumbar puncture, evoked potentials, and magnetic resonance imaging.

POSSIBLE, PROBABLE OR DEFINITE

In classifying the disease, the Poser[415] protocol is used. It takes both clinical and paraclinical information into account. Depending on the number of exacerbations, the evidence of lesions, the symptoms, or the test results of the tests performed, we would speak of: possible multiple sclerosis, probable MS, or definite MS (with clinical or laboratory confirmation).[144]

WHAT IS LUMBAR PUNCTURE FOR?

In the hands of an expert, lumbar puncture should not cause discomfort. It allows us to study of immunoglobulins of the cerebrospinal fluid (CSF) and thereby eliminate many possible diagnoses.

The immunoglobulins are usually found at high concentrations,[363] especially IgG, and specific zones called oligoclonal bands can be seen.[iii] Levels of IgG are somewhat lower in men and in the late-onset and chronic-progressive forms of the disease.[iv]

Immunoglobulin M is not so high (55%), and is related with the activity of the disease: it increases during flare-ups and is higher in patients who have more relapses.[487]

THE PATHS OF VISION

The nerve fibers conduct electrical potentials better if they are surrounded by myelin; when the myelin sheath is missing, conduction is slower. For ths reason, before diagnosing multiple sclerosis, the speed of conduction of the optic, auditory and somatic sensitive pathways is measured.

At the back of the head, near the part of the brain in charge of vision (occipital lobe), we place some electrodes. They will allow us to record the changes in potential produced (evodked) when we give a stimulus to the patient's eyesight. (a flash of light, for example).

These are visual evoked potentials. If they are slower than normal, they indicate that the optic pathway is lesioned, even though the patient may see well and resonance shows normal. Evoked potentials are also very useful in following the evolution of the disease.[319]

If there is optic neuritis on one side, the visual potentials usually show that the other nerve is also affected to some extent.[125] Many multiple sclerosis patients who never had problems with vision may reveal alterations with visual evoked potentials.

This corresponds with the findings of autopsies: the optic nerve is affected in nearly all cases.[125] This test is so sensitive that it can be used as an objective confirmation of the hot water test.[v]

THE PATHS OF HEARING

It is essentially the same wtih the auditory evoked potentials; in this case, with a sound right next to the ear, and the electrode placed over the temporal cortex. Or somatesthetic potentials can be obtained: electrical stimulation of the skin surface, and the evoked potential gathered over the parietal cortex.// potenciales somestésicos:??

A series of waves or changes in potential are registered and, depending on their amplitude (their height on a graph) or latency (how long they take to appear), we can deduce how the visual, auditory or sensitive paths are functioning. In his way, minor alterations that would have gone unnoticed in a routine clinical examination can be detected.

The procedure in not painful at all, has no contraindications, and is very helpful for diagnosis and assessing evolution, above all when optic neuritis is present.

In persons with multiple sclerosis, 75% show altered visual and somaosensitive alterations, and 50% of auditory evoked potentials are altered. (The latter are also called brainstem auditory evoked responses, BAER, because the paths explored cross the brainstem.)[291]

POWERS NO LONGER IN OUR OWN HANDS[vi]

His wife hardly felt a thing again that night, and so the gentleman finally decided to find out if he were impotent.

The neurologist at the day clinic took a little time to have him drop his pants and he tested the cremasteric reflex: he lightly rubbed a wooden spoon against the man's thigh, and the testicle on that side drew up a little.

Later, the bulbocavernosus reflex: upon pressing the glans, the muscles of the penis contracted. The sensitivity on the perineum was all right, and there were no symptoms of incontinnce, so they thought it would not be a case of multiple sclerosis.

It was probably a problem of psychic origin, they commented. But the man had no intention of going to a psychiatrist, so he asked that they do further tests. They told him to come at night to have his erections measured while he slept. There is a simple, logical explanation: if the cause of the impotence is psychological, the subject will be uninhibited at night and will have spontaneous erections.[302]

They placed a device on his penis to measure turgescence and rigidity. He dreamed of his favorite actress that night and got an "A" on the test. When the neurologist gave him the results, he congratulated him and told him the medulla was just fine.

The only other possibility to look into was a problem with the nerves running to the genitals, so he referred him to a neurophysiologist.

THE NERVE OF SHAME

The pudendal nerve[vii] supplies sensitive fibers and motor fibers of the external genitalia (penis and scrotum in males) and the anal sphincter. Using an apparatus called "electromyograph," we are able to objectively evaluate its functioning.

An electrode placed on the penis will emit a mild electrical current and stimulate the dorsal nerve of the penis (sensitive); the potential produced (evoked) can be gathered by a second electrode situated over the bulbocavernosus muscle (at the base of the penis) or on the anal sphincter, which will tend to contract.

The amplitude of the evoked potential and the latency (time between responses) are measured.[300,423,470] It is the most precise test for impotence.[viii]

VITAMIN B12 LEVELS

The concentrations of vitamin B12 in the blood should always be measured when multiple sclerosis is suspected or diagnosed.[435] Macrocytic anemia is frequently found, in association with low leves of B12 in blood and CSF.

A dietetic deficiency in B12 can aggravate the symptoms of MS,[195,554] because this vitamin is necessary for the formation of myelin and immune responses.

Multiple sclerosis begins earlier in persons with a serious lack of vitamin B12.[469]

A GOOD JUDGE DESERVES A GREAT WITNESS[ix]

The judge in the courtroom of multiple sclerosis is the physician. He dictates diagnosis and prognosis, but not only on the basis of clinical criteria. His sentence now leans on the testimony of a special witness: magnetic resonance.

A painless test, involving no complications or aftereffects, which provdes a truthful, objective, and exact testimony of the course of the disease.

Magnetic resonance imaging is highly sensitive: it detects lesions in 90% of the patients it is performed on. The problem is its lack of specificity.

In multiple sclerosis, brilliant periventricular areas are seen in the white matter; however they also appear in other inflammatory or vascular diseases. "Everything that glitters is not an MS plaque"[559]: the hyperintense areas may indicate demyelination, but they also can be indicative of edema, gliosis, or a loss of axons. And so, errors in diagnosis are all too frequent.

RESONANCE IS NOT INFALLIBLE

A normal MRI does not mean that multiple sclerosis can be discarded.

It is diagnosed in over 90% of the cases, but it may also show negative if there are few plaques and they are located in the spinal cord, brain stem or optic nerves[490,527].

In such cases diagnosis must be completed with clinical data, with evoked potentials, and the study of CSF.

In phase T2 of the resonance we see "more lesions" than there really are. The images obtained are less specific and larger in size than the area actually damaged.

They do not accurately reflect clinical incapacity, [47,328] but they are useful in evaluating the evolution of the disease.[390]

RESONANCE WITH GADOLINIUM

In phase T1 of the resonance we can pick up the inflammatory images by creating an intravenous contrast using gadolinium.[329] In this way, we are able to detect "budding plaques" that have not yet given symptoms – a total of up to 5 or 10 times more plaques.[27,204]

This is extremely useful in clinical trials to evaluate the efficacy of new treatments.[331,340] This technique differentiates between "active" lesions and inactive ones; but it may also confuse plaques and merely inflammatory zones.[112]

MAGNETIC TRANSFER IN THE RESONANCE

Magnetization transfer is a new modality[x] applied to imaging in order to obtain higher quality images.[532] More lesions can be seen than with conventional resonance,//MRI, and they are clearer and more sharply contrasted.

The properties[xi] of the lesions can also be assessed, that is, whether they are active or old lesions. That is why it is considered a much more specific test.

DIFFERENTIAL DIAGNOSIS

Multiple sclerosis can be confused with many other diseases[480] which we will merely name here: systemic Lupus erythematosos[302] (the two diseases have been found to occur within a family)[494] primary Sjögren syndrome,[127,355] nodose panarteritis, Behçet's syndrome, AIDS, tropical spastic paraparesis, sarcoidosis,[495] acute disseminated encephalomyelitis, neuromyelitis optica, Lyme disease,[169] cerebrovascular disease, menigovascular syphilis, medullary angiomas[68] or angiomas in the brain stem,[526] paraneoplastic syndromes, apparently tumoral lesions as seen by CAT,[13] heredotaxias, subacute combined degeneration of the spinal cord, myelopathies of unknown origen,[316,515] leukodystrophies, and Arnold-Chiari malformation.[324]

THE NEURALGIA WAS SCLEROSIS

If a young person with no dental problems goes to the specialist with a "trigeminal neuralgia," we must have an MRI done, because it may be multiple sclerosis.[153]

It would be the third most often cause of this condition, after arterial compression in the prepontine area and a tumor pressing on the nerve.[397]

ANOTHER VERSION OF "VERTIGO"

When a person has "vertigo," it is usually traced to problems with the inner ear or the neck. The otorhinolaryngologist ("Eye, ear, nose and throat" specialist) or a traumatologist may therefore be the first to see a case of multiple sclerosis that began with acute vertigo and was diagnosed as acute labyrinthitis.

But in reality, it would been a vestibular neuronitis, only due to the demyelination of the nerve fibers involved.[213,367] The patient improves in the following weeks (spontaneously or with the help of the vestibular sedatives prescribed) and the start of a multiple sclerosis sneaks past us.

THE PARALYSIS THAT CAME FROM THE TROPICS

Immunological alterations in multiple sclerosis resemble those of certain retroviral infections.[xii]

Tropical spastic paraparesis is caused by the HTLV-1[xiii] and occurs in certain regions of the Carribean, Central and South America, India and Africa.[185,235,353,442,443]

Women are affected more frequently, and suffer from paralysis and sphincter problems, at times with sensitive disorders of the legs as well.

It is a chronic demyelination of the medulla[353] with an altered immunological cell response.[235] In endemic areas, tropical spastic paralysis afflicts one in every one thousand inhabitants.[iii] It even resembles MS regarding prevalence. May we be looking at *tropical multiple sclerosis*?

In Japan, a similar myelopathy is produced by HTLV-I. Some affirm that multiple sclerosis, tropical spastic paralysis and HTLV myelopathy are diverse manifestations of one single disease caused by a retrovirus.[262,442]

MULTIPLE SCLEROSIS AND AIDS

Into the doctor's office walks a young man with symptoms of "disseminated affectation" of the nervous system. MRI shows hyperintense lesions with "characteristic" periventricular distribution.

The diagnosis would probably be sclerosis... because he didn't tell us or didn't know that he carried the AIDS virus. So what we see is really a secondary leukoencephalopathy.[523,524]

Some 10% of AIDS patients present an encephalopathy, and the lesions detected with MRI are similar to those of multiple sclerosis, giving way to some mistaken diagnoses.

9. How does the disease evolve?

We do not know how a given case will evolve. Many years ago, when one heard about multiple sclerosis a wheelchair came to mind, because only the very serious cases were diagnosed. Yet there are people with multiple sclerosis who never found out they had it; they die of old age, and the disease is discoverd in the autopsy.

The first exacerbation usually clears up without leaving sequelae. Some patients only experience two flare-ups in all their lives, and they recover well. Among those who have frequent relapses, some improve remarkably and others go on accumulating sequelae until they are incapacitied. There are chronic forms, without flare-ups, in which the patient gets worse slowly but progressively.[490]

THE CHRONOLOGYⁱ OF MULTIPLE SCLEROSIS

A person is born with a certain genetic combination that makes his "immunitary temperament" special. If before age fifteen this individual comes into contact with the noxious external factor (a virus, a certain food or toxin, a specific climate, etc.)ⁱⁱ the immune system is definitively upset and it no longer recognizes the body's own myelin (or certain components of it).

The immune cells (T lymphocytes, macrophages) move through the blood to the cerebrum, cerebellum and spinal cord. At some points, the blood-brain barrier is broken, and the cells destroy the myelin that surrounds the axons. The result is a marble- or cream-colored acute plaque. After a few days, recovery begins, the lesion begins to remylinate to a greater or lesser degree, and the symptoms improve.

Some time later (days, months or years may go by) the process repeats itself, with new lesions (relapses or flare-ups). We do not know if this occurs spontaneously or because the individual comes into contact with an external factor (the same one as before or a different one?).

Generally, the blood-brain barrier breaks at the same sites, but new acute plaques are added.

Eventually, disseminated around the brain and spinal cord there are plaques in different evolutive states: some are acute, some chronic, and others have undergone several processes of worsening and recovery --the "chronic burned plaques". In the latter, the successive demyinations and remyelinations have produced irreversible damage to the axons.[iii]

MULTIPLE MECHANISMS, MULTIPLE COURSES

As the mechanisms are multiple (hereditary, environmental) multiple evolutions are produced.

Some patients present a single minimal episode that leaves no sequelae, others die of old age unaware they had MS, and others, rarely, begin with a copious display of symptoms, quickly get worse quickly, and are soon incapacitated. The disease may take any of these courses, or any course in between.

What is most usual is for the disease to have exacerbations and remissions. A quick flare-up of symptoms appears in a matter of hours or days, lasts some six to eight weeks, on the average, and then goes away slowly, but not always completely.

FOUR TYPES OF EVOLUTION

The many theoretical forms of evolution can be summed up, for practical purposes, as four:

1) In the *benign form* (10% of cases) there are mild, intermittant relapses, with nearly complete recovery..

2) The *relapsing-remitting form* is the most common (40%), with episodes of acute or subacute neurological disorders, followed by periods of improvement and stabilization.

3) The *secondary chronic-progressive form* begins like the one we have just described (RRMS), but then it gets worse little by little, without clear phases of remission, and a gradual accumulation of signs and symptoms is produced.

4) The *primary progressive form:* from the very beginning the disease shows a chronic evolution;[iv] there are no relapses or remissions, the symptoms worsening slowly but inexorably.[144]

BEGINNING AT 27

Multiple sclerosis usually begins between the ages of 20 and 35 [275] (the average is 27).[v] There are some differences between men and women, between blacks and whites, among different latitudes and ethnic groups.

When the disease appears in men or in a geographic region where it is less frequent, the onset is later. As if the key factor setting off MS were not only less frequent under these circumstances, but less efficient as well.[275]

REVERSIBLE STAGE

At first the symptoms tend to be reversible (see Chapter 2). In reality, a process of remyelination takes place with multiple sclerosis, but it is usually incomplete, and progressively reduced in quantity. During the first few years of the disease we can hope that the lesions, and therefore the symptoms, will remit after the acute phase.[341]

AN ATTACK EVERY YEAR AND A HALF

The flare-ups are unpredictable, but statistics tell us that they take place every eighteen months.[441] Many times the first few exacerbations make old symptoms worse, but no new symptoms appear. Young adults have more relapses, one or two per year, and each lasts between four and twelve weeks.

WHY THE FLARE-UPS?

The mystery of the exacerbations lurks in all autoimmune diseases. Vitiligo and psoriasis involve an immune problem, and as they cause lesions on the skin surface, we should be able to relate the flare-up with some factor, right? Yet we are not able to.

In multiple sclerosis it is even harder to attribute the relapses to something definite, and sometimes there isn't even a suspect.[170] Other times there is. The conditions most frequently observed in association with relapses are respiratory infections. Often times the patient reports having had "a cold" [1] one or two weeks before the relapse. This would seem logical in that it could activate the immune system.

Based on this reasoning, the same could happen with some vaccines. Up until now, no one says that multiple sclerosis patients shouldn't be vaccinated because no clear relation has been observed after vaccination campaigns involving large populations.[vi] But medical intuition warns us to keep vaccines to a minimum.

FROM THE FLARE-UP TO CHRONIC PROGRESSION

These are the so-called secondary progressive forms. The patient is used to having temporary exacerbations now and then. But then, after some time, the relapses become more frequent, so frequent that it is hard to distinguish between the relapses and the remissions. And finally, the symptoms spread out progressively, "like an oil slick," with no clear intervals in between.

THE YEAR OF PROGRESS

What year did the relapsing-remitting patient turn into a chronic progressive patient? This is a very important bit of information. It indicates the beginning of a secondary progressive form of the disease, and the prognosis therefore changes.

This unfortunate "year of progress" has a worse prognosis when it is later in appearance. Another negative clue is an accumulation of many exacerbations in the previous months. And the change in evolution is worse for women.[344] If a relapsing-remitting form is going to turn progressive, it tends to do so in the first five years of the disease.[47]

BENIGN AND "SUPERBENIGN" SCLEROSIS

At times multiple sclerosis has a benign evolution. As we said before, some MS patients never even see the doctor. And if they had just one mild episode, there may be no sequelae whatsoever. Approximately

10-15% of the patients have only moderate motor limitations or limitations of another sort after 20 or 30 years.[120] Cases of minimal affectation may be classified as "superbenign" or "hyperbenign."[29]

THEY NEVER EVEN KNEW

And then there are those cases when the first indications of the disease are found in the autopsy of a person who lived a normal life to a ripe old age. They are known as the clinically silent forms of multiple sclerosis. They lead us to believe that the real incidence of the disease is higher than what epidemiologists might tell us.[208] Much higher, according to one study:[497] one hundred autopsies revealed that one or two brains ?? (mean???) had cerebral plaques although symptoms had never appeared. //mucho más frecuente: en cien autopsias, uno o dos cerebros tienen placas de esclerosis múltiple que no habían dado síntomas.

We are dealing, then, with a frequent adverse phenomenon that is generally benign, but able to initiate the lesions of multiple sclerosis in humans, some of whom will evolve poorly.[172]

MARBURG IS A TOUGH TYPE

The other side of the coin. There is one particularly dangerous type of multiple sclerosis, with a serious, acute evolution, that was discovered in 1906 by Marburg.[315] Fortunately, it is rare. Besides the extensive and intense plaques in the central nervous system, an inflammatory primary demyelination appears on the peripheral nerves.[253]

SEVERAL MULTIPLE SCLEROSES

There is not one but a number of multiple scleroses, we could say. At least the disease has very different variants.[508] The genetic base of immunological peculiarity quite possibly varies from one patient to the next. Also varied are the factors that trigger the autoimmune response (virus, diets, or others). And different, as well, are the responses of the immune system: activation of T lymphocytes or of macrophages, humoral reaction, etc.

In the end, the lesions of a given patient are similar to each other, but they are not at all like the lesions of other patient:[vii] in some there is more demyelination, in others a loss of oligodendrocytes, or the axons are affected more. The only conclusion we can come to is that there are different multiple scleroses, different patients or subgroups of the disease, with different pathogeneses.[viii]

BRAIN, SPINAL CORD AND MIXED PATIENTS

There are patients who have more plaques in the brain and others with lesions predominantly in the spinal cord. In the "spinal" patients, the physical incapacity is greater, whereas in the "brain" patients the mental deterioration is more evident. Common sense might have told us, but a controlled study came along to prove it, by comparing clinical exploration, neuropsychological tests and magnetic resonance imaging.[553]

As time passes, a variety of symptoms can be added up: brain, spinal and other sorts, creating a tight *collage*[ix] of sequelae.

TEN STEPS FOR THE INCAPACITY

Each exacerbation is like a rung on a ladder, and the patient goes a bit higher on the scale of incapacity. There are several scales used to measure the incapacity, but the one used most in MS is the Kurtzke scale, which goes from 0 to 10. The average incapacity in a patient who has suffered from the disease for many years is not the same as the patient who has had one or two exacerbations.

For this reason a variate is applied: the incapacity progression index or quotient. Thus, the degree of incapacity on the Kurtzke scale is divided by the years of duration of the disease.[253]

Simply stated, about one third of the patients will have an acceptably comfortable life, another third will accumulate a series of defects that will modify their activities but not prevent them from having a normal family and professional life.

The less fortunate third of patients will witness the progression of the disease and need a wheelchair or special assistance at some point.[441]

YOU CAN'T FLOWER AT FORTY

Multiple sclerosis is a progressive disease; nevertheless, over the years the relapses usually become more distant in time, and less intense, at least insofar as the sequelae left. (The same is true with transverse myelitis or isolated optic neuritis.)

On occasions, the danger passes. Some patients who felt overwhelmed by the symptoms of the disease and things they read or heard about it might end up having virtually no more problems.

After a few years, the multiple sclerosis has "disappeared" from their lives. They are the patients over 40 –over the hill, as some say. They can look back on the previous years that were free from exacerbations and breathe a deep sigh of relief. Or repeat the famous words of Lucrecio, later borrowed by Lord Byron: *Suave mari magno.*[x]

THE "MARK" OF SCLEROSIS

There are persons who carry the "mark" of the disease yet never have symptoms. A genetically predisposed individual has contact with that unidentified factor that alters his immunological system. He thus acquires a distinctive stamp or trait that makes him susceptible in the future to multiple sclerosis ; that is, if other favoring factors are there, or the protective factors are absent.

The "mark" of sclerosis is a special clinical or subclinical situation that is systemic, meaning it is not restricted to the nervous system. It is a general immunological disorder, but its main effect is to make the blood-brain barrier more vulnerable to a variety of agents that can make it more permeable.[409]

This modification o the BBB has been confirmed using neroimaging techniques. It is non-specific //of unspecified origin ¿?? (it may have to do with a virus, a vaccine or a traumatism), but it constitutes a prerequisite for multiple sclerosis. Other factors will be determinant in the actual appearance of symptoms. This "pre-MS" has been found in identical twins, when only one of the two actually develops the disease.

CHILDREN WITH MULTIPLE SCLEROSIS

It is unusual for multiple sclerosis to begin in childhood (before age 15). Magnetic resonance imaging may show a child to have certain "alterations" of the white matter that do not necessarily represent MS. Besides using the Poser criteria, other neurometabolic and neuroinflammatory diseases capable of causing demyelination at an early age must be considered.

When produced, sclerosis in children has a more acute onset (tumors or encepahalitis may have been suspected at first) and there is a greater inflammatory component than in adults. It is more frequent in girls than in boys, and tends to begin with only one symptom, generally of a sensitive or sensory type. Recovery from the exacerbation can be rapid, but afterward evolution is slow, relapsing and remitting,[115] with a risk of becoming a more serious chronic progressive form. In children who begin with optic neuritis, an external triggering factor is usually identified. It may be an infection or vaccination.[xi]

MULTIPLE SCLEROSIS AFTER 50

One´s first reaction should be of disbelief if confronted with a case of MS that began after age 50. If it is the real thing, most likely the onset was earlier but went unnoticed. The differential diagnosis must look principally for vascular diseases that produce demylinating lesions (for example, multi-infact ¿? encephalopathy).// (encefalopatía multi-infarto y otras)[22].

FROM BIRTH TO OLD AGE

Summing up the life story of multiple sclerosis: a child is born predisposed, but disease-free; in puberty she acquires the disease, but is symptom-free. The adolescent begins with symptoms that get worse in adulthood to a varying degree. In old age the disease settles down and its progression is negligible.

10. A strategical neurologist

It was the weekend, and the young college student woke up early to study for Tuesday´s exam because she wanted to go out that evening. The night before she had noticed a tingling sensation on her face. Now she felt it even stronger. And when she got up to walk, she staggered as if drunk.

Five days later, parties and exams are far from her thoughts. She is in the hospital, unable to move her legs, and a young doctor is asking her for details about that "cold" she had two years back, when she lost her eyesight temporarily. Since she had bounced right back to normal she hadn´t believed it to be important.

But now it matters. She doesn´t know yet what is wrong, but it must be something serious, so sudden... her life might never be the same again. She is scared. She thinks she heard someone mention sclerosis, but she's afraid to ask, unsure whether she really wants the doctors to be frank with her.

WHEN THEY TOLD ME, MY BLOOD RAN COLD

Telling someone they have multiple sclerosis causes a great impact.[i] It is a point of transition that requires tact and time. Here is where the strategic know-how of the neurologist comes into play.

The situation must be presented with sensitivity, taking the patient's character and psychological standpoint into consideration. The neurologist should be clear when giving the diagnosis and deciding what plan they will adopt –together—to improve things.

STRATEGY[ii] AND TACTICS FOR TREATMENT

In different individuals, different immunopathological mechanisms are at work. For that reason, it is not surprising that they may react differently to treatment. Medication that is useful in one patient may be ineffective in another.[341]

Depending on the type of evolution, the neurologist, like the chess player,[373] will distinguish strategy –long-term treatment-- and tactics: specific actions taken when problems arise, for instance a flare-up, a pregnancy, or an operation.

DESIDERATA[iii]

What would be best for the patient can be summed up as these four ideals, published in 1970:[59]

1. complete recovery
2. prevention of relapses
3. keeping the incapacity from getting worse
4. ensuring that treatment(s) will be less harmful than the disease.

IS IT OR ISN´T IT A FLARE-UP?

A flare-up is produced by a new plaque of demyelination, or by the reactivation of an old one. By definition, to qualify as a flare-up or relapse a new symptom should last more than one day, and be separated by more than a month from the previous exacerbation..

A pseudo-exacerbation (false flare-up) has nothing to do with the activity of the disease. It is produced by other problems that aggravate the neurological symptoms of the already existing plaques. For example, if the patient has a fever or has been in a hot atmosphere (a hot bath, a very warm room, or under the sun), he or she may feel worse, yet it does not constitute an exacerbation, because they are better as soon as the temperature goes down. Likewise, spasticity of the legs may be more bothersome when it coincides with a urinary infection or is associated with other types of discomfort.[496] But it is not a flare-up.

HOW OFTEN TO THE NEUROLOGIST?

That depends on the type of multiple sclerosis. In benign forms, one visit per year is enough, and it can be a short one. In patients with several exacerbations per year, or with a cumulus of sequelae, more visits are logically needed, and the neurologist will take more time with them. Also needing extra time are patients participating in treatment trials, those requiring psychological assistence, and those with a special treatment or complicated device (for instance, the baclofen pump).

JUST WHAT AWAITS ME IN THE FUTURE?

All multiple sclerosis patients ask the neurologist this question, directly or indirectly. No one can make any sure claims about how the disease

will affect a certain person over the next few years, but there are statistical data that may serve as a general guideline.

The general prognosis is not as bad as one might think: nine out of ten patients have long intervals with no or very few troublesome symptoms;

one in three is still practically free from sequelae years after the onset of the disease; and three out of four patients stay active and independent for many years after diagnosis.[290]

"THE SECOND FLARE-UP" AND "THE 5-YEAR RULE"

They are two medical oracles. If the interval between the first and second exacerbations is long, the disease will be more benign.[253] Bear in mind that the patient may not have been aware of the initial manifestation of the disease (perhaps years earlier), and his first trip to the doctor may be with the second flare-up.

The rule of five years is quite reliable The situation in which the patient finds himself after five years with the disease helps us predict the evolution of the following ten years. If there were infrequent exacerbations and limited sequelae, the course will be benign; or the reverse will be true.[496]

Incapacity at the five-year point is roughly three-fourths of what it will be ten years thereafter (15 years after diagnosis).[253] In other words, a patient gets just about as bad as he is likely to get during the first five years; the next ten will affect him, too, but to a lesser degree. In the natural evolution of the disease the trend is for the relapses to get milder and less frequent.

HOW LONG DO I HAVE TO LIVE?

The thread of the Moiras[iv] is ten years shorter for multiple sclerosis patients, but this is an average figure that shows many variations. The life expectancy after diagnosis is from 25 to 42 years (to be added to the patient's age at diagnosis). It is worse for the forms with a cerebellar onset. [60,399,400,414]

Some 80% of patients are alive 25 years after diagnosis (more women than men in this group), which is somewhat lower than the life expectancy of equivalent populations[557]. If we bring statistics up to date, it would be more than 25 years, because we are now diagnosing patients at earlier and earlier ages, and so they live longer after the diagnosis.

The disease in itself is not mortal; but secondary complications may bring on death. If we avoid them, the patients will enjoy longer lives. In particular, we must guard against bronchial pneumonia due to the aspiration of food particles or fluids (take care at meals), decubitus ulcers, urinary infections (pyelonephritis and uremia), and falls.[311,312] Recent advances in treatment make life expectancy improve steadily.[60]

BAD AUGURIES[v]

Again we are dealing with general statistics,[60,400,437,545] but, all in all, the factors associated with a worse prognosis are:

- The male gender: the disease is less frequent in men, but its evolution is worse;
- Onset with vertigo or cerebellar symptoms, with psychiatric disorders or multiple symptoms;
- When paralysis or tremor are important, or urinary problems are persistent;
- "Family" forms (more than one family member is affected) or forms that are progressive from the start;
- Late onset forms: the first manifestations come after age 40 and gait is affected more, usually signalling a progressive course of the disease;
- A short interval between the first and second exacerbations;
- Altered visual evoked potentials on both sides;
- Patients who respond poorly to corticoids.

GOOD AUGURIES[vi]

They are only statistics;[252,400,440,545] but in general the following cases have shown a better evolution:

- Women: though more often affected than men, the disease is usually not as serious in females;
- Onset with sensitive symptoms, optic neuritis, diplopia (double vision);
- Quick recovery from the symptoms (in less than six months);
- The relapsing-remitting forms that begin in young adults (but not in childhood);
- A long interval between relapses (most importantly, before the second exacerbation; if more than a year has elapsed, it's a very good sign);
- A good response to corticoids.

New drugs are the best of auspices. In the past there was no treatment for multiple sclerosis, and nowadays the neurologist has to decide between several different treatments (which we will have a look at later). For starters, which interferon do we choose?

THE INTERFERON OF DISCORD

Discordia was the very picture of envy as she tossed an apple asking Paris to take it and to give it to his favorite of three goddesses.[vii]
The neurologist has to make a similar decision regarding the therapeutic strategy for the patient to follow.

Interferons are substances that react with antibodies.All the new drug treatments are good, but which one will best prevent the progression of the disease in our patient?

- Interferon beta-1b was the first to come out, and more studies attest to its efficacy. It is given subcutaneously three times a week.
- Interferon beta-1a is more recent, and therefore its effectiveness is not as well documented. It is given intramuscularly once a week (there is also a subcutaneous version???) // (ahora sale también subcutáneo)
- Or... we wait for copolymer (available in some health centers) in Spain.

To help make this decision, we should study Chapter 13: Interferon and new therapies.

11. The flare-up and other emergencies

Multiple sclerosis follows a long and winding road. It evolves in a chronic form, or a chronic-relapsing form, but there are also emergency situations, such as the acute flare-ups that require urgent corticoid treatment.

"CORTICOID" COMES FROM CORTEX

The suprarenal glands,[i] true to their name, are situated above the kidneys, and furnish the body with certain hormones. In their internal zone (suprarenal medulla), adrenaline is made, while in the external zone (suprarenal cortex), corticoids are produced.

On occasions, the brain[ii] secretes another hormone, ACTH (adrenocorticotropic hormone), which stimulates the suprarenal glands so that they will produce corticoids. If we want a patient to have more corticoids, there are two possibilitites: giving her synthetic ones, or injecting ACTH so that her suprarenal glands will manufacture more natural corticoids.

ACTH AGAINST RELAPSES

In 1951 we began to use ACTH to treat the exacerbations or relapses of multiple sclerosis.[154,174] Instead of giving the body foreign corticoids, it seemed more natural to inject ACTH so that the patient could increase production on her own. Significant improvement was observed, and in 1970 a thorough study[448] cleared up therapeutic doubts: ACTH (and therefore corticoids) improved the symptoms of acute flare-ups, including optic neuritis and other diffuse manifestations of multiple sclerosis.

EASY-TO-USE CORTICOIDS

ACTH has two drawbacks: it must be administered by injection, and, more importantly, we do not know exactly what dosage is needed, because that depends on the response of the suprarenal cortex of each patient. Corticoids (also called corticosteroids) are easier to use, and their efficacy in treating relapses is just as good or better.[392] Injectable corticoids allow us to give high doses safely. There are also tablets and drops, which make it easier for the patient to continue treatment at home.

WHATEVER YOU DO, DO IT SOON[iii]

What is important about corticotherapy is that it be initiated as soon as possible. Its efficacy is greater if administered just before or during the inflammatory phase of the disease. Among other actions, corticoids diminish the inflammation of the nervous tissue, besides halting the activity of the immune system, which is altered.[iv]

GIANT DOSES WORK

Kibler[255] had rabbits with "artificial" multiple sclerosis;[v] he gave them corticoids in proportion to their weight,[iv] and they remained just as ill. He increased dosage: double, triple, ten times, twenty times the correct dose... and they improved. Then he dared with patients suffering from acute flare-ups of MS. They were injected 200, 300,

500,. and up to 1000 mg a day. The results were so positive that "megadoses" became generalized. (we also refer to them as // ¿?? los denominados "pulsos" de corticoides,) //as a safe, effective treatment.[219]

At present, we treat acute flare-ups with large doses of methylprednisolone (500-1000 mg) diluted in an introvenous serum that acts slowly (one hour). Depending on the evolution, these megadoses can be given for three to seven days. Then the dose of corticoids is decreased progressively, orally, for three or four weeks. In patients treated with megadoses the cognitive functions also improve, as demonstrated using evoked potentials and adequate verbal stimuli.[146]

AFTER THE BATTLE, THE WAR GOES ON

Thanks to corticoids, the relapse was shorter and left fewer sequelae. We won the battle, but the disease is still there. What will happen next? In the coming years, will the patients treated with corticoids do better than those who were not given drug therapy?

An if corticoids are good for the exacerbations, why not give them more frequently? These questions are difficult to answer, because conclusive studies are needed, but we may put forward a few criteria.

THE OPTIC NEURITIS RINGS TWICE

If we treat an acute optic neuritis with corticoids, vision returns quickly. It is one of the clearest indications of corticoid action. But some believe that, in treated patients, there is a greater risk that the optic neuritis will recur in the future.[38]

CORTICOID ADDICTS

In the final analysis, corticoid abuse produces serious damage: gastric ulcer, psychosis, septicemia ("blood poisoning"), decalcification of the bones, and suprarenal insufficiency. And even worse, the patients who use take corticoids for long periods of time get "addicted": that is, when the medication is discontinued, new exacerbations appear.[256]

A MEGADOSE EVERY OTHER MONTH

So what do we do when there are no flare-ups, but the disease progresses slowly and steadily? Corticoid megadoses have been recommendended even for these chronic forms,[549] but treatment cannot be continuous.

A new study involves therapy with short (3-5 days) megadoses of corticoids given every one to two months, which are then discontinued suddenly (not gradually reduced with smaller oral doses). The idea sounds all right, but we still do not know what the long-term results will be.

PREVENTING THE SECOND FLARE-UP

What usually happens is that the multiple sclerosis is diagnosed at the second or third exacerbation. But let's imagine that the neurologist was really on the ball and after the first exacerbation we must acknowledge the fact that we are dealing with a demyelinating disease. Should we wait? Can we do something to avoid or delay the second exacerbation?

Let's have a look at statistics. Among optic neuritis patients we find that, two years later, 16% of the untreated patients have developed multiple sclerosis, as compared with 14% of those who took corticoid tablets (prednisone or similar). However, we see less than half (7%) as many cases among those who were treated for their optic neuritis with intravenous megadoses of corticoids.[38] The conclusion is obvious: optic neuritis should always be treated with corticosteroid megadoses.[vi]

DEATH BY SUNNING

She was a 35-year-old woman with relapsing-remitting multiple sclerosis. She went to the beach and lay in the sun for too long. Her body temperature went up and she was overcome with fatigue. Though she was moved to a cool place, the muscle weakness continued to get worse, and death was imminent.

A true, fatal case that has been published.[203] It is a rarity, but we tell the story in order to insist on the risk that prolonged exposure to sunlight entails for these patients. It is a potential emergency that is easily avoided. The neurologist or general physician should remind their MS patients about it before they go off on summer holidays.

12. Protect us from our defenders

The doctor will try to dismantle the defense mechanisms of the patient with multiple sclerosis. It is not really such a strange prospect, in the context of auto-immune diseases: the agents that usually protect us (T lymphocytes, macrophages, etc.) misidentify the enemy, and instead of fighting against foreign germs, they attack the myelin of their own neurons. Their immunity has a masochistic tendency, we could say, and it has to be stopped. So we intervene with immunosupressants, drugs that are able to debilitate tha natural defenses of the organism.

As we saw earlier, exacerbations of multiple sclerosis are treated with corticoids because these act to suppresss certain natural immune mechanisms. We will now describe nonspecific immunosupressants, which all too frequently give contradictory results and lead to numerous secondary problems.

PREGNANCY AS A NATURAL IMMUNOSUPRESSANT

The fetus is strange yet well-received entity, and if the mother does not expel it it is because her defenses are somehow diminished. Pregnancy, then, is a natural immunosupressant state, a sort of allotransplantation in which tha paternal antigens are provisionally admitted by the mother. Indeed, during gestation there are fewer exacerbations of multiples sclerosis; it is afterwards, during the puerperium, when the disease gets worse (see Chapter 7).

THE GOOD AND EVIL OF AZATHIOPRINE

Azathioprine[i] inhibits all the organism's defenses: it blocks the production of lymphocytes and antibodies. In the long term, it offers some improvement of MS symptoms (the number of flare-ups and degree of incapacity are slightly decreased). Scanty benefits that do not compensate for the multiple drawbacks: azathioprine lowers the number of leukocytes in the blood (leukopenia), is toxic to the liver, and may cause nausea, fever, or skin problems.

Even so, it is used as a prolonged treatment (2-3 years) in selected cases (young patients, secondary progressive and short evolution forms).[39,40,144]

CYCLOPHOSPHAMIDE AND HAIR LOSS

In order to avoid psychosomatic problems, serious clinical trials are "blind" (the patient doesn't know what medication he is taking) or "double blind" (neither the patient nor the doctor knows).[ii] This is impossible to do with cyclophosphamide because persons taking it lose their hair, vomit, and pass blood in the urine.[517] The supposed benefits do not make it worthwhile. Better to avoid it.

WHEN REMEDIES ARE WORSE THAN THE ILLNESS

In treating multiple sclerosis, many immunosupressants have been used. It is difficult to explain to patients that statistics "seem" to show that there is some improvement with a drug treatment that the patient has been taking faithfully for two or three years. What they notice is that they feel worse when they take the medication.

- Cyclosporine does damage to the kidney, the liver, raises blood pressure and increases the risk of cancer.

- Cladribine is a potent antilymphocyte agent used in treating leukemia and lymphomas. Some adverse results have made researchers interrupt the clinical trials that were underway.[40,519]

- Methotrexate is used in rheumatiod arthritis; it may cause fibrosis or cirrhosis of the liver and pneumonitis.

IMMUNOSUPPRESSANTS ON THE WAITING LIST

Immunosuppression relies on drugs that are more and more specific and less toxic than in the past. The following "newcomers" appear promising, but conclusive studies are needed.

FK506: a powerful immunosuppressant used in organ transplants.[40]
Sulfasalazine: used for intestinal autoimmune diseases (such as ulcerous colitis or Crohn's regional enteritis).[519]

Mitoxantrone: it has a strong antitumoral activity, and lower myocardiac toxicity than similar molecules.[519]

THE RISE AND FALL OF CHEMOTHERAPY

Chemotherapy will be with us for a number of years, still, but its use is clearly on the decline.

The new techniques of immunosuppression, which are more specific and less harmful, will substitute many of the drug therapies now available.

REMOVAL OF ANTIBODIES BY CHANGING PLASMA

Plasma is the fluid portion of the blood, which contains, among other things, antibodies. Since we assume that multiple sclerosis patients have antibodies that act against their own myelin, it would seem logical to remove their plasma and exchange it for artificial plasma (with no antibodies).

This procedure is called plasmapheresis, and it is also employed in other autoimmune diseases such as myasthenia // (gravis??), when we know that the patient has antibodies against the receptors of his muscle fibers. Notwithstanding, in multiple sclerosis no specific autoantibody has been identified yet, and the results of plasmaphersis are not clear.

We do know that it is a complicated, costly procedure that entails certain risks (infection, the failure of some organ).[211] It is hardly ever performed nowadays.

FLUSHING OUT THE BAD LYMPHOCYTES

This treatment is founded on the same principle. If the lymphocytes attack the myelin, they ought to be changed.

The procedure, called lymphocytapherisis, consists of extracting a great quantity of lymphocytes from the patient. It is even more expensive than plasmapheresis, and the benefits are equally uncertain.

IRRADIATING THE BAD LYMPHOCYTES

A similar idea for eliminating the harmful lymphocytes, this time by applying radiation. A total irradiation of the lymphoid zones is carried out. It seems to provide some benefits in chronic progressive forms of MS.[90] But other findings raise doubts, and the untoward effects are quite serious.

ALIEN GLOBULINS VS. OWN ANTIBODIES

Normal subjects also have a certian tendency to develop autoantibodies, but they get rid of them by attacking with some substances called anti-idiotypes. They circulate in the blood within the great group of immunoglobulins.

If we obtain nonspecific immunoglobulins by mixing the plasma of thousands of healthy subjects, there will be a multitude of anti-idiotypes. If we then transfuse the immunoglobulins to patients with multiple sclerosis (or other autoimmune diseases) the anti-idiotypes should, in theory, stop the activity of the antimyelin autoantibodies. This is the premise that researchers are now working with, and the preliminary results are promising.[2,40,109,132,133,499]

MONOCLONAL ANTIBODY "MISSILES"

This form of selective immunosuppression is based on an ideal: the artificial development of antibodies that selectively destroy the components of the immune system that are causing trouble –be they cells, substances or lesser elements). Like a guided missile.

13. Interferon and the new therapies

We can try to improve the long term evolution of multiple sclerosis with nonspecific immunosupressors. We now have "immune-modulators," new treatments for modifying the immune system in a more selective manner.

Interferons and copolymers are the two best known immunomodulators, but we will mention some other new treatments as well.

INTERFERING WITH NEW INFECTIONS

If a virus invades a cell, something happens to prevent that cell from being infected by other agents afterwards. It is like when Rome invaded Greece: Athens, already subjected, was no longer afraid of the Persians, their age-old enemy. "Romanization" was a disagreeable new situation for the Greeks, but one that at least interfered with other invasive attempts.

We see something similar (to put it simply) in the cell invaded by a virus: it produces a substance that "interferes" with other viruses and protects the cell from subsequent infections: interferon.

GOOD AND BAD INTERFERONS

Interferons are special proteins (glycoproteins) that are produced by the cells of the organism[i] after they are infected by a virus. There are more than 20 varieties: interferon alpha, beta, gamma, and others, etc.

In theory, all of them are good for the normal person, because they will defend him from other viruses. But in multiple sclerosis and other autoimmue diseases, some are damaged, such as interferon type II (gamma), which increases the number of exacerbations. [ii]

Type I interferons (alpha, beta, omega and tau) are the most important for resistance to other viruses. It was discovered that they helped improve mice wtih experimental allergic encephalitis (the animal model for multiple sclerosis),[58] and have since been given to MS patients. We can think of them as the "good" or "useful" interferons.[454]

ARTIFICIAL (RECOMBINANT) INTERFERONS

It takes great amounts of time and money to obtain natural interferons in the laboratory. The solution came along in the 80's, when recombinant DNA technology became popular and it became relatively easy to clone the genes of interferon and its products.[398]

It has meant a real revolution. We can now derive "artificial" varieties of interferon, and they can be applied to other immune or viral diseases.

MULTIPURPOSE INTERFERON ALPHA

Interferon alpha can be used successfully for a cold[111,206] or for some kinds of encephalitis.[558] It provides improvement in some types of hepatitis (non-A, non-B) but can be damaging in others (autoimmune hepatitis).[388]

INTERFERON BETA-1b

It is a recombinant (artificial) interferon obtained from a bacteria (*Escherichia coli*). It is unlike natural interferon beta in the composition of two of its aminoacids and in the fact that it is not glycosylated . It was the first interferon on the market (Betaseron), and it is used every other day in subcutaneous injections, which allows any patient with a bit of training to administer it on his or her own.

The pilot study[228,229] shows, without a doubt, that interferon beta 1b reduces the number and intensity of the exacerbations in relapsing-recurring multiple sclerosis:[iii] patients treated with high doses had one third fewer flare-ups.

But the most spectacular results were seen with magnetic resonance imaging: two years later, examinations with activity data dropped to half their former values, and the total number of active plaques was reduced by no less than 83%.[393]

Interferon beta-1b also improves cognitive functions.[404,405]

FEWER AND MILDER FLARE-UPS

In patients treated with interferon beta-1b there are fewer exacerbations, and they are less intense. It seems that final incapacity is also improved, but to a scarcely significant degree if we use the classic evaluative scales (EDSS). The reason might be[392] that, in the long run, the clinical deficit and the incapacity do not depend on the primary inflammatory processes, but rather on secondary or independent factors: the loss of axons and gliosis, which would be responsible for the symptoms.

MRI TAKES THE STAND

Magnetic resonance imaging is the best witness of how the disease is coming along, and one important research group has determined its testimony to be unequivocal:[393,230] interferon beta-1b is beneficial in three ways:

1) The untreated (control) patients had twice as many new lesions as the treated patients.
2) In the patients treated with interferon beta-1b there was a reduced thickness of the periventricular alterations (which are thought to determine the progression of the disease).
3) Interferon beta-1b continued to be effective five years later.

No one doubts, after seeing the MRI results, that treatment with interferon beta radically changes the pathological anatomy of multiple sclerosis: there are fewer new lesions and they are smaller, above all in the periventriaular areas, which are the ones associated with a poorer prognosis.

HERMENEUTICS[iv] OF MRI

With magnetic resonance imaging we see fewer and smaller lesions. We could logically assume that things are better than they were. But has the disease really improved? Or has it only been delayed? Will it get worse as soon as treatment is discontinued? Why hasn't the incapacity of the patient improved more if there are fewer lesions? What might happen ten or twenty years from now to these patients who seem to be responding well?

These and other questions[328] depend on the results of upcoming clinical trials. For the moment, we cannot answer them. Better we remain cautious and keep an open mind when interpreting what is "evident."

WITNESS FOR THE PROSECUTION

After five years monitoring treated patients, no serious complications were seen. But not all the evidence goes in favor of the interferon beta. It can give rise to some minor problems: a sort of "cold" syndrome, local reaction at the site of injection, analytical alterations and a worsening of depression (with the lurking possibility of suicide attempts). In addition, neutralizing antibodies may be formed over time.

THE NOVICES CATCH COLDS

When they start treatment with interferon, half of patients (52%) show signs of a "common cold": runny noses, red eyes, and some may have fever, muscular aches or cramps. It is the rite of initiation.

Soon they get used to the treatment, and after two months only one in ten still "has a cold," with milder signs now. The patient may feel some relief if we raise the dosage of interferon beta more slowly, or if we associate ibuprofen[392] or pentoxifylline.[545]

INJECTION SITES AND ANALYSES

The site where interferon beta was injected may appear reddened or hardened, and at times there is even a local necrosis of the skin. Blood analysis shows lower leukocytes or slightly higher hepatic enzymes. In three or four months, these values spontaneously return to normal, ant the patients haven't noticed.

DEPRESSION AND SUICIDE

Some patients treated with interferon beta 1-b have had severe depression, on occasions with attempted suicide. We must be very alert to this possibility, even though the depression may be previous to treatment, from having to face a chronic disease. Tolerance can be improved with anti-depressants.[348]

It appears that those who have more cold-like symptoms also get more depressed.[230] With interferon beta-1a depression is not found to increase. Con el interferon beta-1a no se ha encontrado que aumente la depresión[234,364].

NEUTRALIZING AN ALLY

The interferon that we inject into a patient is her ally. But her immune system doesn't know that. It sees the interferon as something foreign (actually, it is an extraneous protein) and, with time, tends to destroy it by producing antibodies that will neutralize it.[v]

Some 35% of patients treated with high doses of interferon beta produce neutralizing antibodies against the drug,[231] nearly always during the first year and a half of treatment. In these patients, the drug gradually loses effectiveness,[vi] and the results are, of course, poorer – almost the same as in the placebo group (the persons in the study who were given an inert substance instead of the real thing). On the other hand, the patients who did not develop neutralizing antibodies evolved much better.

EPHEMERAL CONSENSUS

Clinical trials are one thing, and what happens in clinical practice is another. There was a meeting of experts to discuss and come to conclusions about how to use interferon beta in the context of everyday doctors' offices.[305] Guidelines were established about how to administer it, and to what type of patients. In some countries these guidelines are follwed to the letter to keep health costs down.

But, as we gain in knowledge with the results of new studies, continuously underway, we must modify our criteria, most often in a more liberal direction. For example, in the past we could not prescribe interferon beta for the progressive forms. But look what happens...

IT WAS UNETHICAL TO GO ON WITH THE STUDY

We already knew that interferon-beta was useful in relapsing-recurring forms, but its use was not approved for progressive forms because no one had demonstrated its effectiveness. Till one day a trial was begun with progressive multiple sclerosis patients who were divided into two groups at random: some were given interferon-beta injections, and others were injected with an innocuous liquid, a placebo.

As the study went on, the treated patients improved considerably, so much that it was truly unfair to leave the other group at a disadvantage. It was unethical to carry on with a study that prevented the placebo group from reaping the benefits of interferon beta. So the experiment came to a halt and interferon was given to all. Interferon beta is not only good for relapsing-recurring MS, but for the progressive forms as well.

INTERFERÓN BETA-1a

It, too, is a recombinant interferon, but it is not obtained from bacteria; it is elaborated from genetically manipulated mammal cells (from the ovary of the hamster). It is glycosylated//a glycosyl and is identical to human interferon. It recently became available commercially (Avonex??). Published studies and studies still underway point to optimistic results.

It is the first drug that has reduced –moderately, yet with statistical significance— the progression of MS in some patients with the relapsing-remitting form. The reduction in annual relapses also proved significant, and very similar to that observed with interferon beta-1b.[234]

It offers the advantage of being given just once a week, intramuscularly. Among adverse effects, the initial pseudo-cold symptoms were also reported, but the local reactions at the injection site were lesser, and cutaneous necrosis was not observed.

DEPRESSION DID NOT GET WORSE

Unlike beta-1b, interferon beta-1a does not appear to augment depression and suicidal tendencies. An improvement in cognitive functions has been documented. Moreover, the production of neutralizing antibodies is limited.[339]

APPEALING COMPARISONS

Soon there will be more, but for the moment there are three beta interferons: Betaferon ¿?(beta-1b, subcutaneous, every other day), Avonex (beta- 1a, intramuscularly, once a week), and Rebif (beta-1a, subcutaneously, three days per week). The methodology of the preliminary studies of each did not coincide: the degree of incapacity of the patients, the dosage and the parameters for following treatment were different.

Not all comparisons are ugly; some are desirable. We are awaiting the results of the most recent experimental studies with similar designs in order to decide which of the beta interferons is best for a given patient.

A REVOLUTIONARY CHANGE

The introduction of the three beta interferons has meant a revolutionary change in our approach to treating multiple sclerosis, at both a clinical and an anatomopathological level.

Things will never be that same for multiple sclerosis patients; their future now holds real promise. With our present knowlege, we can say that all patients with sclerosis should be treated with interferon beta.

INTERFERON GAMMA: THE BAD GUY

We all produce interferon gamma naturally, and at first it was used as a treatment for multiple sclerosis. But the patients got worse, not better,[vii] and testing had to be stopped.[387]

Actually, the good results from interferon beta are due, in part, to the fact that it blocks some interferon gamma actions. A new treatment strategy for multiple sclerosis is oriented toward obtaining new drugs capable of blocking the sinister interferon gamma.

GET USED TO EATING MYELIN

Multiple sclerosis patients do not tolerate their own myelin. In order to get them "accostumed" to it, less sensitized to it, we can make them eat a bit of myelin.

This notion is similar to the one behind antiallergic "vaccines": progressive doses of pollen or dust are given to allergic persons so that they will eventually stop reacting. A touch of poison can heal, states one homeopathic principle.

It works in lab animals: if given myelin orally, a tolerance is produced, preventing experimental allergic encephalitis. Human tests have been done with complete oral myelin,[217] or with a portion thereof, the so-called myelin basic protein (MBP), which is administered by injection.

COPOLYMER, A MYELIN SIMULATOR

We can take this idea a little further, and give a bit of antigen to "desensitize" the organism, to create tolerance, but now more selectively.

Copolymer-I (glatiramer) is a mixture of synthetic polypeptides that resemble the myelin basic protein (Copaxone). They contain four natural aminoacids (glycine, alanine, lysine and tyrosine), just like those in myelin,[167] and they compete with myelin when the autoantibodies come along.

This leads to a rise in suppressor lympthocytes, and the immune response to the myelin basic protein comes to a halt. This is a vague description, because the precise mechanism at work is not yet fully understood.[171]

TWO FOR THE PRICE OF ONE

Copolymer I and interferon beta have additive effects, and sometimes synergystic effects, in supressing the alterations that the myelin basic protein produces in vitro.

Both drugs are expensive, but they may work together; some are already proposing their combined use in a single patient.

LINOMIDE AND THE KILLER LYMPHOCYTES

Everyone's body contains killer lymphocytes, They are natural defense agents that are highly aggressive, and they are less plentiful in persons with autoimmune problems.

Linomide (Roquinimex) is a drug that, given orally, stimulates the production of the necessary killer lympoocytes.[viii]

It has been tested in relapsing-remitting multiple sclerosis, and in chronic MS. Imaging shows fewer lesions, and incapacity improves. But testing has been postponed because of the risk of cardiac complications (pleuropericarditis).[1,14,250,519]

A LA RECHERCHE DE LA MIELINE PERDUE

In search of the lost myelin, if Proust[422] will excuse me: that is where some of the new therapies are directed. Is it possible to recover or replace the myelin that was destroyed?

Research is focused on three horizons:

1) growth factors (insulin-like growth factor I)[298]
2) oligodendrocyte transplants, that would form new myelin, and
3) autoantibodies.

GROWTH FACTORS

Growth factors are substances similar to hormones that facilitate the repair of the destroyed myelin. They may represent a completely new road to treatment.[82]

In multiple sclerosis, the oligodendrocytes regenerate part of the destroyed myelin, but at a slow pace in comparison with the speed at which it is lost. It is hoped that the growth factors can accelerate and intensify the remyelination process —enough, at least, for the symptoms to improve.

Some experiments with animals have given positive results: for instance, IGF-1 (insulin-like growth factor 1), which promotes the proliferation of the precursor cells of oligodendrocytes.[ix]

GLIAL CELL TRANSPLANTS

Different forms of transplanting are being tested using the cells derived from the glia:[114] are being tested: cells from the oligodendrocyte line, "immortal" cell lines,stem cells, Schwann cells and xenogenic transplants.

We are far from obtaining practical results.

AUTOANTIBODIES

Autoantibodies are being tested to see if they can contribute to remyelination in one of two ways: through a direct mechanism (the autoantibodies stimulate the oligodendrocytes or cells that favor them) or indirectly (the autoantibodies inhibit pathogenic immunologicl processes).[342]

NEW SCALES FOR NEW THERAPIES

The new therapies –interferons and copolymers—reduce by one-third the number of relapses, and the lesions produced are shown by magnetic resonance to be less extensive. It would be logical to conclude that incapacity is also reduced, but that has not yet been demonstrated.[253]

As we said earlier, comparisons can be positive. That is why the two types of interferon beta are now being compared –to each other, and to the copolymers and the classic immunosuppressors.

The patient and his or her family are relatively less concerned about the number of relapses, or what resonance tells us about the number of lesions.

What matters most to them is whether the degree of their incapacity increases or not, and the scales habitually used do not tell them enough in this sense. The latest evaluative studies are paying more attention to parameters that assess life quality and cognitve state; the latter is a crucial factor in the patient's daily social context and work-related activities.

14. A solution for every problem

Multiple sclerosis can be treated, though there is not yet a cure for it. Besides treating and preventing exacerbations, we can improve many symptoms and alleviate specific problems or discomforts. There are everyday troubles that might seem trivial (to the docotor) but that the patient considers very important because they affect the quality of his or her life. They trust that we help them solve these difficulties.

Some remedies were already given in relation with psychic changes (Chapter 6) or problems involving sex or sphincters (Chapter 7).

IMMOBILIZING SPASTICITY

When the pyramidal tract is damaged, patients have problems of spasticity. The muscle tone augments, making the joints get stuck in fixed postures, and hindering movement of the extremities, especially the lower ones. The spasticity, even when mild, reduces mobility and does damage to the joints. It is to blame for most of the troubles and incapacities these patients face. The physiotherapist knows how to exercise the joints and help align them correctly.

Often the spasticity is accompanied by hyperreflexia and clonus (the tendinous reflexes are exaggerated and sometimes prolonged). Then it truly is laborious to do something as simple as getting up from a chair: the legs are rigid, and on attempting to rise, the excess of reflexes spoils the movement with involuntary oscillations that increase clumsiness.
If we train the patient to execute movements in an adecuate order and manner, very positive results can be achieved.[290]

DRUGS FOR SPASTICITY

There is a fixed spasticity (which immobilizes permanently) and episodic spasticity (appearing as painful spasms from time to time). Baclofen (Lioresal) can be used to fight either. It is a drug with a central action, and is usually taken orally. In complicated cases, a perfusion pump is used.

Dantrolene acts peripherally, inhibiting muscular contraction. It is very useful for painful cramps, but it diminishes muscle strength and is better restricted to use in a hospital setting. Threonine is sometimes effective in these cases.

RELAXATION WITHOUT WEAKNESS

Tizanidine (Sirdalud) reduces medullary reflexes and also acts on the brain. It debilitates to a lesser degree than baclofen, although it may produce nausea or dryness of the mouth. Tetrazepam, which is milder, also has fewer side effects; it is said to have the best benefit/risk ratio.[394]

Gabapentin[i] is a recent and surprising discovery. In reality it is an antiepileptic drug, but using it at low dosages alleviates spasticity, and it has practically no untoward effects.[362]

I CAN'T WALK WITHOUT THE SPASTICITY

At times, we manage to suppress the spasticity and the patient comes back to tell us that he has even more trouble walking. His legs are weak, and the increased muscle tone of spasticity was precisely what helped keep them rigid, enough to hold him upright. In such cases it is not adviseable to reduce spasticity too much.

KILL THE MESSENGER

The "messenger" of the spasticity is the peripheral nerve (which is healthy). Although the lesion is located in the brain or spinal cord, it is the nerve that carries orders to the muscle to contract excessively. Without nerve impulses there can be no spasticity; so one possible treatment is to block them.

Let's use an example. Some patients have a very tiresome way of walking, known as "scissors gait," with the thighs close together owing to the spasticity of the adductor muscles.

The excessive contraction is due to a lesion in the spinal cord, but the "messenger" is the obturator nerve. By blocking the nerve with injections of phenol,[ii] the spasticity is completely suppressed and gait improves.

We may also exercise action on other nerves that transmit spasticity: cutting the medullary roots (dorsal rhizotomy), or stimulating the spinal cord (with electronic devices). And there is one very effective alternative: relaxing the muscle directly, wtih injections of botulinus toxin.[545]

RELAXANTS AND ANTI-INFLAMMATORY AGENTS

Relaxants have less of an antispastic capacity, and anti-inflammatory agents none at all, but both improve the sensation of rigidity, as well as other bothersome sensations. Diazepam (Valium) is a good muscle relaxer, but relatively high doses are needed, causing drowsiness.

FATIGUE AND MUSCULAR WEAKNESS

Fatigue leaves one incapable of carrying out daily chores. It is recommended that the patients avoid heat and take intermittant rests; exercise is needed, but the patient must know when to stop, before getting tired. Cool showers help, and the room temperature should be kept low, if necessary with air conditioning.

Sometimes tiredness is alleviated with amantadine or pemoline.[265] The effectiveness of 4-aminopy... is being tested for fatigue and weakness: la 4-aminopidirina[iii]: it blocks the potassium channels, prolongs the duration of the action potential and may improve conduction in demyelinated neurons.

AGAINST TREMOR

The tremor in multiple sclerosis is usually of the "cerebellar" type; that is, it prevails when voluntary movements are executed. We can try to improve it with a range of drugs: clonazepam, propanolol, isoniazid, acetazolamide, and the aforementioned gabapentin. In difficult cases, steriotaxic surgery may be required, implanting a deep-seated stimulator in the thalamus.[551]

NEURALGIAS AND OTHER PAINS

The trigeminal neuralgia and other painful disturbances are treated with carbamazepine or gabapentin.[222]

Chronic neurogenic pains are more difficult to treat. Conventional or major analgesics may be combined (orally or intrathecally), or tricyclic antidepressants (amitriptyline) or transcutaneous nerve stimulation can be used.

CAN MEMORY BE IMPROVED?

Some try to improve memory and other cognitive functions through mental exercises and compensating strategies (see Chapter 15). Others use nootropic medication (cyticoline, pyracetam) with irregular results. Patients with cognitive deficits improve with interferon beta-1b (Betaseron/Betaferón)[404,405] , and even more significantly so with intramuscular interferon beta -1a (Avonex).[iv]

PSYCHOLOGICAL DISTURBANCES

If depression is noteworthy, it must be treated. Fluoxetine, sertraline or paroxetine may be used. Some patients taking interferon beta-1b get even more depressed, and special care must be taken with them. If the low state of spirits persists, change to another treatment: interferon beta-1a (Avonex) or copolymer (a totally different molecule).

CAROB FLOUR TO SWALLOW

Some patients have trouble swallowing liquids. If we thicken them just a bit, the liquids go down much better. There are derivatives of carob flour that are tasteless and practically calorie-free. Different consistencies can be obtained, depending on the amount added: syrup, gelatin, or purée.

UNDERGARMENTS FOR INCONTINENCE

Incontinence can make life very difficult for the patient, above all when outside the home or traveling.

When treatment has proven unable to solve the problem, the only alternative is to cover it up: there are special undergarments designed with additional deposits (in Spain their ancient name is "martingalas"[V]). They may be particularly convenient to wear when on a trip.

FLYING WITH A WHEELCHAIR

Needing a wheelchair does not preclude air travel or other means of transportation. There is always a mode of access for persons with special needs; it is not a favor or preferential treatment, but simply the acknowledgement, more and more widespread nowadays, of the rights of people with handicaps.

It is better to plan ahead, though, and contact the travel agent or the airlines to decide the conditions in which the passenger will travel.

15. A good general physician

The neurologist designs the treatment strategy for his multiple sclerosis patient. But the daily battle with the disease must be faced by the patient with his family doctor, whom he has known for years. He will be the patient's mentor[i] or guide for the problems that come up, or for suspecting an exacerbation and sending the patient to the specialist.

The GP or family doctor diagnoses 5% of the cases of multiple sclerosis, and he is consulted between 15 and 20 times per year on the average, mostly on account of problems with sleeping, incontinence or urinary infections.[110]

CLOSE CONFIDENCES

The multiple sclerosis patient goes to the neurologist from one to six times a year, depending on the case. But he needs someone close to confide in, a good general physician who understands her, who is well informed about her neurological situation, who knows enough about multiples sclerosis, and who can solve everyday problems.

When the time comes, too, this family doctor should be capable of determining whether the patient's complaints signal a new flare-up.

THE TERRIBLE DOUBT OF THE APPEARANCES

The patient is overwhelmed with anxiety at the prospect of suffering another relapse. She wonders every time she feels something that reminds him of old symptoms, or when a new discomfort or disturbance appears. Above all when they are subjective annoyances, such as tingling, or when they are very transitory, such as a slight difficulty with vision.

"Is this a new flare-up? This is the same sort of tingling I felt when they made the diagnosis of MS." The terrible doubt of appearances[ii] hangs over her. She's not sure whether to go to the neurologist, or perhaps start taking corticoids on his own.

In dealing with a disease with such varied and unpredictable symptoms, any modification of well-being produces insecurity. The general physician of an MS patient has one very important function: he must be able to distinguish a flare-up from other complaints. This diagnosis is fundamental. It should be done with certainty, and relaying that confidence to the patient. In the case of an exacerbation, or of a lingering doubt thereabouts, the patient will be referred urgently to the neurologist. But many unnecessary visits to the specialist can be avoided if the GP knows just how to differentiate between a real relapse and the state of apprehension of a patient with worrisome symptoms.

THE PERIOD WAS MISTAKEN FOR A RELAPSE

Do not confuse it with a flare-up: there are women with multiple sclerosis whose symptoms get worse before their menstrual period. It is one more finding that points to the relation of the disease with the endocrinal system.

On these days of the cycle there are abrupt changes in the levels of sexual hormones and endogenous opioid peptides, and plasmatic melatonin fluctuates; this produces an increased neural excitability and immune alterations.[462]

BLOOD, SWEAT AND FEVER

Even though it is not a relapse, a multiple sclerosis patient may get worse for some minutes or hours.

It may be that metabolic by-products have accumulated in his blood, owing to kidney or liver insufficiency, or he may have anemia or an infection.

Or perhaps the patient is sweating too much and gets dehydrated because it is too warm in the room, or he has just taken a hot bath. It may be a fever brought on by anything from a common cold to a urinary infection. Sometimes a patient breathes very quickly (hyperventilation) because he is tired and nervous.[290]

IATROGENY AND PRECAUTION

The general physician should oversee the short term problems associated with some medications. Tricyclic antidepressants can cause urine retention, muscle relaxants and sedatives increase weakness, and 4-aminopyridine can cause convulsions. In the long run, the GP will watch out for the osteoporosis that can be brought on by corticoids, and he will do periodic urine analyses to check the number of leukocytes in patients taking immunosuppressants.

And contrariwise. He will avoid the sudden interruption of certain drug treatments. A brusque drop in corticoids can aggravate MS symptoms; taking away antidepressants suddenly may lead the patient to despair, and discontinuing baclofen can trigger the appearance of hallucinations or agitation.

PREVENTING THE URINARY INFECTION

It is elementary. Urinary infections are very frequent in multiple sclerosis patients, above all in those with a great amounts of residual urine (they have trouble with miction and the bladder tends to get too full).

Some need a catheter from time to time, and it must be done with adequate hygienic measures. Other times the infection is not acute, but chronic.

The patient with a urinary infection may not notice problems with his urine, complaining instead of general lack of well being: she is weaker or more tired than usual, has a bit of a fever, has lost her appetitie. The generaly physician must be one step ahead of the problem and have urine cultures run on these patients on a regular basis, even in the absence of complaints. When an infection is discovered, the germ must be identified before prescribing the most appropriate antibiotic.

AN ACIDIC FLOW

The better the urine flows, the fewer chances there are of infection. If incontinence is not a problem, the patients should be urged to drink lots of liquids. And of course, obstacles such as bladder stones or obstructions of the neck of the bladder must be eliminated.

Bacteria prefer alkaline environments. Therefore, we can combat them by acidifying the urine with vitamin C, or increase fruit intake (cranberries are very good).

OUR DAILY BOWEL MOVEMENT

Some older persons are obsessed with having a bowel movement every day, and the general physician should convince them that it is not always necessary. In multiple sclerosis, constipation is a frequent problem, but many patients are fine if they defecate every three or four days.

Diets rich in fiber are good for all of us, but in particular for multiple sclerosis patients. If there are no bladder problems, plenty of liquids can be recommended as well. At times, fecal softeners or peristaltic stimulants may be needed. Other times there may be blockage due to compact feces that will require enemas or direct manipulation.

Not all intestinal troubles are because of the MS. Some of these patients already had celiac disease (gluten enteropathy), colitis or idiopathic constipation. If doubts remain, a radiological study with a contrast medium will unveil a "lazy" intestinal transit or an anal-rectal dysfunction.[370]

THE NEUROLOGIST DOESN'T UNDERSTAND ME

The general physician often hears comments from the patient about the specialist. *"The neurologist says that I'm better, but I'm not, I'm worse."* This discrepancy in the results has been objectified[iii] and has its explanation[452]: the specialist pays more attention to clinical and complementary tests. After a treatment (be it with corticoids, interferon or chemotherapy), he notes improvement in the reflexes, or on the Romberg test or auditory evoked potentials. But the patient is not concerned about test results: she feels nauseated, or just worse in general, and that hampers her daily routine. The quality of life is what matters to the patient.

Under these circumstances, the general physician, being closer to the patient, can help a lot; it is he who directs the general aspects of care that call for the collaboration of nurses and other medical assistants.[321]

DAILY FATIGUE

We cannot repeat it often enough: one of the prime symptoms of multiple sclerosis is fatigue. The patient gets very tired, and not because of the paralysis or depression. We do not yet understand the mechanism, but there is an organic factor –not an imaginary one—that makes the patients more prone to fatigue.

The general physician, who sees the patient regularly, should give this symptom the attention it deserves: it is one of the most incapacitating factors. It should not be brushed off; nor, on the other hand, should it be confused with an exacerbation. The GP can recommend rest, staying out of the heat, and avoiding rich or large meals.

PAINFUL OSTEOPOROSIS

In chronic multiple sclerosis, both immobilization and the repeated corticosteroids contribute to a process of osteoporosis that may prove to be quite painful. It must be prevented, through clinical check-ups and diagnosis with imaging techniques, together with adequate exercise and calcium supplements.

PRESSED NERVES

If a person is immobilized, with osteoporosis and weight changes, his peripheral nerves may be damaged, simply because the body positions maintained keep some body parts pressed against the crutches, the wheelchair, or the bed. The general physician should be specially attentive to signs of lesion of the median nerve in the wrist or of the peroneum of the knee (from the straps of the leg braces).

ACUTE ABDOMEN FROM MS

The "acute abdomen" is one of the most frequent emergencies that the general physician will have to attend to. If a patient with multiple sclerosis presents abdominal pain, distension, vomiting and constipation, the suspected cause will be in the spinal medulla (a new flare-up or a deterioration of the neurovegetative motor regulation) [301].

MIELINA SANA IN CORPORE SANO

There is no certainty about what might speed up recovery of the myelin after a relapse, nor what can be done to avoid or appease the arrival of another. Common sense, however, tells us that a good general state of health is the best defense against any disease.

The myelin will be better protected in a healthy body, and the general physician will watch that his patients keep good, nutritional eating habits (a balanced diet), that they stay physically and mentally active (without overexerting themselves), that they avoid stress, and that they promote their own personal independence as much as possible, while staying integrated in society. And finally, he will ensure that they themselves are knowledgeable about all potential complications, so that they can be prevented.

Needless to say, factors that would make the symptoms worse (heat, fever, dehydration, anemia, infections and other illnesses) must be avoided.) [290].

ADAPTING TO LIMITATIONS

Adaptating to one's limitations and instrumental devices, be they leg braces, crutches, or a wheelchair, may require some psychological support. It can be done in different manners, depending on the neurological disease that necessitates it. In patients with multiple sclerosis, an emotional adaptation is observed: introverted but stable.

The style of adaptation is somewhat worse than in patients with medullary lesions who adopt an attitude of "problem solving." But those who are poorest at adapting are patients with cranial traumatisms.[548]

SNUBBING NATURAL DISGRACES

We all undergo the trials and tribulations of aging, illness, and the progressive loss of capabilities. To know thyself is indispensable. We must be aware of the good and bad that can surface at particular times, and program our activity bearing them in mind.

Some people get more wrinkles, others put on more weight than they would like to. Many people need glasses, crutches, or wheelchairs; and hearing aids or dentures are going to be necessary sooner or later.

We have to face the adverse circumstances of nature and life. Take the advice of Gracián,[186] *"laurear el natural desaire"*, coping with negative circumstances by finding a way around them. Julius Caesar, determined to conceal his baldness, made wearing a laurel fashionable![iv]

THE GP-SPECIALIST SYNAPSE

The trend in modern-day medicine is to knock down hurdles between primary and specialized attention. The patient with multiple sclerosis will reap the benefits if, besides confiding in his general physician and his neurologist, he helps the two keep up a frequent and cordial relationship, promoting the interchange of data and opinions about his clinical situation. Other specialist, in Urology, Lungs, or Digestion, may be needed as well.

16. Four rehabilitators

In multiple sclerosis, we need four "rehabilitators," that is, four levels attention and action:

- Rehabilitating the body
- Rehabilitating the soul
- Social rehabilitation
- Rehabilitation of the home.

In order to rehabilitate the body, physical therapy is needed, attending to muscles and joints, language and mental functions. The rehabilitation of the soul calls for acknowledging stress in order to combat it, adapting one's lifestyle, and keeping channels of communication open in the family and social circles. Rehabilitation of the home means adapting it to the needs of the patient to make his daily activities easier (occupational therapy); simple, imaginative resources an be used, or else the latest technological advances

REHABILITING THE BODY

Specialists agree that motor rehabilitation is fundamental, but some don't insist on this enough when they talk with the patient. Arthrosis ¿? and muscular atrophy ¿? lie in waiting of these patients with limited mobility, and the only way to elude them is through active and passive rehabilitation. Techniques used at present include novel aspects that are, of course, adapted to this disease in particular.

Equally necessary is muscular rehabilitation. Postural instability and locomotor disturbances involve the atrophy of a special kind of muscle fibers (type II) ¿?, which can recover with properly directed physical exercise.

MUSCLES, MIND AND ENJOYMENT

Physical activity is a great means of alleviating tension. During exercise, endorphins are produced. These are natural tranquilizers that relax the body physiologically. Moreover, the muscles, in exercise, are strengthened and stretched. Stretching is important for increasing articular mobility.

Physical exercise, understood as recreation and enjoyment, is also a way of lending some spiritual virtues to the body: energy, daring, patience.[i] "Aerobic" type practices lift the spirits as well as boosting cardiovascular and pulmonary functions. Exercise regulates appetite and sleep, and contributes to a feeling of all-around well-being (NMSS Living) The patient can swim, walk, or use an exercycle or rowing device//static rowboat. Avoid getting to the point of fatigue.

BICYCLES ARE FOR AUTUMN

Bicycles are not just for kids. Even in the autumn (and winter) of our lives, bikes or mo-peds develop neurological circuits that are wasted in persons who won't leave the secure confines of four-wheel vehicles. Remember those thin, agile –physically and mentally—older folks who rode a bike all their lives? For years they developed muscular and nervous networks that integrated balance with visual and spatial perception. Not to mention the physical activity.

Bikes afford a type of psycho-motor rehabilitation, with special attention to the circuits of equilibrium. Patients with multiple sclerosis who can ride a bike (careful with accidents!) can improve their coordination or help prevent future problems.

LEARNING TO WALK

The physician and the physical therapist will offer a critical analysis of the patient's motor capacity and possibilities. They study her potential strength, how the spasticity is reflected in her posture, and the situations that are more likely to produce falls. With this information, they design a strategy for the patient to learn to walk and move around in her daily activity. They will also recommend adequate footwear, braces or other accessories, as needed.

ORTHESES, PROSTHESES AND TECHNOLOGY

To correct fixed postures, or to compensate for the weakness, we can turn to splints and braces or prostheses.[ii] A dropped foot ¿??// pie caído needs a common splint. Deviations//curvature ¿?? of the spinal column call//s for an orthopedic corset, which should not be worn for very long periods.

But even though shoes with reinforcements and canes or crutches are still used, modern technology has provided new resources for persons with motor sequelae.

These are tools invented to serve mankind, just like the watch, eyeglasses, or the automobile, and the patient should not hesitate to use them. The old-fashioned wheelchair can be fully motorized now, or even automatized//robotized. There are numerous new devices designed to facilitate a variety of everyday tasks or activities.

EXCHANGE THE MAGNIFYING GLASS FOR A PC

If optic neuritis left sequelae, the visual deficit can be compensated, to a great degree, using the wide range of possibilities offered by computer technology. A personal computer is more versatile than a magnifying glass. We have scanners, screens of various sizes, and all sorts of programs that can be helpful. With minimal "computer know-how" the patient can gain access to books or other texts, adjusting the size and the background of the screen to optimize visibility..

OPAQUE LENS INSTEAD OF THE EYEPATCH

Diplopia (double vision)[iii] has nothing to do with the eye *per se* (vision also depends on the optic nerve). The patient sees double when the two eyes, poorly coordinated, give respective images that are not properly superimposed.

We can make amends by covering up one eye. Instead of doing this with the old "patched" glasses, which are not very esthetically pleasing, we can use a special contact lens with an opaque center, which blocks the vision of the altered eye. (Check it out on Internet, at http://aspin.asu.edu/msnews/ medres.htm.)

FROM SPEECH THERAPY TO CYBERLANGUAGE

Difficulties with speech are addressed by the speech therapist. He will prescribe specific rehabilitation exercises or techniques, with the difficulties of the individual patient in mind. Again, computers can come in very handy. There are programs that pick up one's voice and allow a person to "write" without hitting a key. Other programs can transform the voice, making it more audible or easier to recognize for others. Patients with disarthria (difficulty in articulating words) or with a voice tremor can use these systems to be better comprehended.

REHABILITATING THE SOUL

Rehabilitation of the soul, the psyche or one's attitude toward life (call it what you will) is crucial in any chronic patient, and especially so in those suffering form multiple sclerosis. We must work on mental capacity, stress factors, family relationships, and social integration (including work or unemployment, associations, Internet, etc.).

MIND-SET AND LIFE QUALITY

No one will deny that it is necessary to rehabilitate the mental functions damaged by a traumatism or brain hemorrhage. Well it has also got to be done in multiple sclerosis. If these patients have a cognitive deficit, life is not so pleasant or easy. Life quality is at stake.[431]

The brain has a certain degree of "plasiticity"; and with adequate training, the areas that remained perfectly functional can take over some of the altered functions. Though not all experts believe in their effectiveness, mental exercises and methods of cognitive "reinforcement" do exist. We can also resort to compensatory strategies[279] to improve overall performance. Healthy people use them too: making task lists, sticking notes on the refrigerator, using an agenda, mnemonic devices, etc.

STRESS AND SICKNESS

We know for a fact that stress can play a part in exacerbations of multiple sclerosis,[189,190,253,542,543] but each individual perceives stress differently. There are situations of real danger that some face serenely, while others get terribly upset if a dish breaks. The mode of interiorizing or outwardly expressing stress varies from person to person as well. Some individuals who seem tranquil are really distressed on the inside. How we feel about daily events can be more important than the events themselves.

LOCATING STRESS

If we are going to attack the enemy, we will have to pinpoint his location first. Anxiety has a very negative influence on many personal capacities or potentials. The first step is to identify the sources of stress in our patient, that is, the situations that produce physical or emotional tension for him in particular.

Once the origins of stress are located, therapy will consist of avoidance or progressive deprogramming, in learning to relax, and in programming positive compensating activities. Self-control techniques are an indispensable part of anti-stress rehabilitation.[314]

IT'S ALL OVER NOW BABY BLUE

So sang Bob Dylan when his marriage came to an end. Separations, like other stressful situations, can trigger a relapse or affect the progression of the disease. Divorce favors multiple sclerosis, and multiple sclerosis favors divorces.[64] But we can't give up. We must urge the patient to rebuild his or her life, and some good may even come of it. After all, life is a garden of forking paths. (Jorge Luis Borges could have told us that.[56])

REDEFINING BONDS WITH ONE'S SURROUNDINGS

Psychotherapy can help improve a situation of abandonment, solitude, and depression where these patients are led by age, illness and other circumstances. One's outlook on life must be readjusted. The way a person experiences illness often reflects his or her way of living. A patient can learn to be more accepting, redefining connections with her environment.

Modern rehabilitation is geared toward social integration. There are even groups of musical therapy for persons with multiple sclerosis.[294] If we manage to "get the patient involved" in her surroundings, some improvement will be evident. Anything that represents achievement or enjoyment will be beneficial.

IN THE BEGINNING THERE WAS ACTION

Depression can be remedied with action. According to Goethe, the usual translation of the book of Genesis, "In the beginning there was the Word," is incorrect. In the first part of *Faust*, he inquires about the true meaning of "Logos," and deduces that it should not be interpreted as "Word" but as "Action."

Action is the foundation of life; life is action. A man is the sum total of the things he has done. Do and act: it will keep depression at bay.

FROM THE *ZOON POLITIKON* TO THE CULTURAL ANIMAL

Another tricky translation, this time of the words of Aristotele. When he speaks of man as the *"zoon politikon"* and we read it as "man is a political animal," we run into some confusion. The philosopher did not mean that all men should get involved in politics; he was merely insisting on the need for men to be part of civic life, in the activities of his city (*cívic* comes from city, and *polis* is the equivalent of city).

Social integration is vital for our patients. For better or for worse, "man is a social-cultural animal." This is increasingly true as our society advances. An individual loses part of his identity when adapting to a new cultural structure, and this gives him a new sense of reality.[iv]

His socio-cultural projection depends on the degree of satisfaction that our patient feels. And this, in turn, depends on whether he is accepted by family and friends, and on his possibilities of working or being an integral part of his environment.

The poorer the psychosocial integration of a patient, the greater the physical incapacity, and this is particularly evident among women with multiple sclerosis.[562]

INTERNET AND SOCIAL CHANGE

Until not long ago, humanity had two basic systems of communication: the press and the telephone.[v] Now Internet comes along: a third system that is interactive, truly reciprocal. It is analogous to the telephone, but not limited to two persons; it adds a common context, a "community" that, unlike classical media, is not generated by specialists, but by the participants themselves. Lévy, the philosopher, describes it as a collective interchange with no control center.[296]

Internet can be used to the advantage of chronic patients, especially MS patients, because they are young and maintain a good intellectual level . From their homes, they can keep up on scientific breakthroughs progress. But what is most important is that they are no longer isolated. Their opinions form part of a community of persons affected by the disease who demand social and medical changes. This weighs on government policies in support of the ill, can contribute to research, and finally, may speed up the arrival of new treatments.

MULTIPLE SCLEROSIS ASSOCIATIONS

They exist in all the more developed countries, and constitute a an enormous aid for patients. They are a sort of union of patients who lay claims to their rights and see that they are respected. In Spain, the AEDEM stands out (Asociación Española de Esclerosis Múltiple), along with the FEDEM (Federación Española de Esclerosis Múltiple).

Nearly all the industrialized nations have similar groups, with strong organizations, independent or collaborative research projects, journals, support groups, and newsletters on Internet. *National MS Society, The MS Foundation, The Federation of MS Therapy Centres, MS Information Source, MS Society of Canada, The Australian State MS Societies, Esclerosis Múltiple Argentina, MS Society of Great Britain and Northern Ireland, Polish MS Society, The Myelin Project, International MS Support Foundation,* etc.

UNEMPLOYMENT AND MS

Multiple sclerosis is the most frequent cause of neurological deficits in young adults. This fact cannot be forgotten when we talk about unemployment, a problem that affects 80% of these partients. Obviously, a patient with some deree of deficit will also be hindered in some ways (réemora[vi]), but he must try to overcome it to improve as a person and be useful to his family and society.

THERE IS MORE TO LIFE THAN WORK

The race of men is condemned by nature to work. But one day the gods took pity on men, and as a respite from their sufferings, they gave them as joyous companions the Muses,[vii] Apollo and Dionysus.

This affirmation comes from Plato,[403] in his *Laws*: we have many possibilities of deriving pleasure and compensation for our efforts: arts are inspired by the Muses (from dance to music and poetry), Apollonian beauty, or Dionysian indulgence,[viii] aside from other sources of delight. This is leisure as the Greeks understood it —time dedicated to cultivating the arts and life's pleasures. In the patient with multiple sclerosis, in any ill person, the search for pleasure should continue. It is the brighter side of *Il dolce far niente.*[ix]

SERVICE DOGS

Trained dogs are very useful, from both social and psychological standpoints, and can help keep the cost of care down.[10] Every patient should have one.

REHABILITATING THE HOME

The house also needs rehabilitating. It costs very little, when you compare it with the huge benefits it provides for the patient, to renovate the living space so that daily activity is easier. This is known as occupational therapy.

There are construction guides and special improvements designed for handicapped persons. Bars or railings in the bathroom or along the walls, changes in lighting, no-spill tumblers to drink from, special eating and cooking utensils. The bed, or the whole bedroom for that matter, can be adjusted to suit the patient's capacities. There are telephones with special devices for dialing, and a ramp or a motorized elevator system could replace steps. The toilet is too low for some patients, and raising it is simple. The height of steps can be reduced with wooden "landings" that take up half of each step. With the right fixtures and a remote control, we can turn on and off lights, the television, or the coffemaker. The whole idea behind technology is to make life better and easier.

A PRESCRIPTION FOR AIR CONDITIONING

We neurologists should have special prescription pads for air conditioners. Our multiple sclerosis patients who live in warm climates really need them as much as any other therapeutical measure. Then, the air technician could go to their homes, draw up a plan, and install as many fans or vents as needed. I'm not joking: one of the most effective treatments available for multiple sclerosis is home air conditioning. Fatigue, such a common complaint, improves considerably.

PUBLIC RESOURCES AND SOCIAL ASSISTANCE

What would be ideal is to have access to persons specializing in this sort of workmanship, and have public funds to cover the costs, after consultation at a patient association (whose influence is on the rise).

Many countries budget substantial economic resources for the home assistance of persons with some sort of deficit or handicap. It is more cost-effective than treating them at hospitals, and the patients themselves are more satisfied. There are volunteers, or persons paid by an institution, who can help patients in their everyday atasks

17. *Alimentum sanum in corpore sano*

The health of the body is forged in the office of the stomach, said Don Quixote[74] four centuries ago. Many people still believe it, and some say that what you eat can prevent or worsen multiple sclerosis. The diets that we will see here are not "miraculous," and their therapeutic efficacy has not been demonstrated. But they ensure proper nutrition, so they can't hurt.

FATS: A SEVENTIES FAD

Myelin contains a special fat --phospholipids. The most popular theory in the 70's was that the type of fats we eat can influence the appearance of multiple sclerosis. Fish is good, but other animal fats increase the risk of MS; there are more affected persons in the countries with greater fat intake.[11,32,45]

THE DEAD WERE FOND OF FATS

Just recently they published a study that had been done before I was born.[510] In 1949, 150 patients with multiple sclerosis were advised to adopt a low-fat diet (less than 20 grams of fat per day). Half followed the advice, the other half did not. Researchers waited 35 years to see the results.

Those who had followed the diet were better off, and after all those years, only 30% were deceased. But not too many of the "disobedient" patients lived to see the day of the last check-up: one in five (80% mortality) had survived, albeit with serious incapacitaties. The conclusion is clear: saturated animal fats aggravate multiple sclerosis, and even moreso in women.[510,511]

ESSENTIAL FATS AND MYELIN

Mammals need to eat two types of essential fatty acids –linoleic and alpha-linoleic— because without them they could not build their own polyunsaturated fats (large-molecule fatty acids, made up of the others).

The diet of western civilization relies heavily on margarine (with hydrogenated fats) and previously oxidized ("bleached") flour. This means to a relative deficiency of linoleic and alpha-linoleic acids that might provoke multiple sclerosis.[i] In these patients, the white blood cells and platelets have less linoleic acid,[152] and its blood level[ii] during a flare-up is even lower.[45]

EATING LIKE ESKIMOS

Fish protects one from multiple sclerosis, because it is rich in unsaturated fats.[365,509,512] Our elders are not likely to forget how, as children, they had to take cod liver oil "to stay healthy." Despite its awful taste, it may have, indeed, kept them safe from multiple sclerosis.

Eskimos do not have MS, and they eat fish almost exclusively. It gives them high levels and a wide variety of polyunsaturated fats (timnodonic and clupanodonic fatty acids).

According to one large study carried out in Great Britain, patients who took fish oils had fewer and less intense exacerbations, although the statistical significance of the results was low. It may not be the tastiest of diets, but it is healthy, inexpensive, and possibly effective in preventing multiple sclerosis.[490]

SARDINES FOR DEPRESSION

The fatty acids found in "blue" fish (tuna, mackerel, sardines, etc.) have anti-inflammatory properties and prevent circulatory diseases. In addition, if these fish oils are lacking, the depression sometimes associated with multiple sclerosis, puerperium or alcoholism can intensify.[216]

Treating depression with sardines is no guarantee of psychological recovery, but it helps and is healthy.

WONDERING ABOUT COW'S MILK

Drinking lots of milk increases the risk of multiple sclerosis, say some. Combining the studies of 27 countries, suspicions arose surrounding cow's milk,[iii] as its intake appeared to be related with the frequency of the disease.[4,313] Cream and butter have minor correlations; cheese and other dairy products have no influence.

THE MYELINATING BREAST

Cow's milk may be bad, but mother's milk is not. Children who were breast fed show a rapid cerebral myelination[97] that makes them resistant to demyelinating diseases in adulthood.[iv] It was recently proposed that maternal nutrition –during gestation, that is-- might also play a role. (The interpretation of results would depend to some extent on a family's socio-economic level.)[44,402]

THE MEDITERRANEAN DIET: FROM MYTH TO RITE

The "Mediterranean diet" is a myth that was first narrated very far from the sea. In an underground laboratory at the University of Minnesota, they discovered the culinary advantages of the lands bordering on the Mediterranean sea. And it now seems that what matters is not (just) what we eat, but how we eat it. A piece of toast with olive oil or a glass of wine will do more good to a Greek than to a Swede.

On the island of Crete, in Rome or in Malaga, bear in mind that besides the dishes, there is a distinct life philosophy in the background: the climate, the sun, the pleasure taken in having a meal together, savoring it slowly. We have an attitude towards eating that surprises foreign visitors.[55] The mealtime ritual is more important than its ingredients.

RICH KIDS EAT MEAT

Upper social classes have more cases of multiple sclerosis.[343,401,438,536] Some relate this finding with the patterns of social conduct,[v] and others with the unique eating habits of children from wealthy families.[42] They consume more proteins (meat in particular) and many foods with chemical additives. Moreover, their "nutritional status" does not waver as it might among the poor.[282,283,286,288]

AND THE CHINESE EAT RICE

In Asia the diet revolves around rice, whereas in many warm climates the staple is corn. Wheat and rye (which, unlike rice and corn, contain gluten) are eatern more in colder lands, by Norse or Anglosaxon populations. Someone eventually associated this with their predisposition to multiple sclerosis, and a new treatment was established: the gluten-free diet. The only cereals[vi] allowed, of course, are rice and corn.

ALLERGIC TO SUGAR OR TOBACCO

And then there are those who think that multiple sclerosis is brought on by a kind of allergy to tobacco and to sucrose or its derivatives. Not only is smoking forbidden; all sorts of sugars must be eliminated from the diet (from sugar beet, cane, molasses, dates...) The strictest proponents of this diet avoid the glycol compounds commonly used in food products or cosmetics. They would turn down a shampoo with glycerine.

CACTUS JUICE

Scientists call these spiny plants from dry soils *"Aloe vera,"* but we also know them as agaves. Their bitter liquid portion contains high concentrations of vitamins, aminoacids and minerals. It was tried as a treatment for multiple sclerosis, and some say it helped. It is a good dietary supplement, though it may cause diarrhea.

EXTRA CALCIUM, MAGNESIUM AND VITAMIN D

A group of young people with multiple sclerosis followed a diet enriched with calcium, magnesium and vitamin D. After two years, they had had less than half the exacerbations statistically expected.[175] The authors of the study attribute the good results to the role of calcium and magnesium in improving the development and structure of the myelin, making it more stable.

NITRATES, NITRITES AND ADDITIVES

In ancient times, cooks only had natural vegetable colors. Around 1700 they began to be replaced with nitrates (especially chile saltpeter), which gave meats an appetizing look and helped conserve them.

In the 19th century, sugar was added. This reduced the nitrates to nitrites, chemically active agents. Some say that since then colorectal cancer, multiple sclerosis and rheumatoid arthritis are on the rise.[285]

THE GEORGICS, OR NATURAL FARMING

In the *Georgics*, Vergil describes the traditional methods of working the land,[vii] quite different from modern farming with artificial fertilizers, chemical pesticides, and transgenic seeds.

Some think that modern agriculture is to blame for multiple sclerosis and other diseases. We don't know; but the fruits and vegetables that the Latin poet ate were surely sweeter and healthier.

MEAT AND MILK FROM BUCOLIC HERDS

The pastors that Virgil describes in the *Eclogues* (also known as the *Bucolics*) did not spoil the milk and meat of their charges with hormones or processed feed.[viii] But modern breeding relies too heavily on artificial substances that detract from the quality of their products and the health of consumers. Some suspect that what animals eat can play a part in multiple sclerosis or other pathologies, and recall that "mad cow disease" did not exactly begin with green grass.

EVERS LIKES IT RAW

Dr. Paul Evers has been treating multiple sclerosis patients in Germany for many years. He believes that it, and other diseases, are caused by the systems of food production and processing. Dr. Evers insits his patient eat fresh foods, preferably raw, as natural as possible.

There are three basic rules:[194] 1) Eat lots of vegetables (including sprouts and fresh and dried fruits) while avoiding animal fats. 2) The fats that are consumed should preferably be unsaturated. 3)Keep daily calorie intake low.

THE WRITER WHO WROTE HIMSELF A DIET

Roger MacDougal is a writer with multiple sclerosis. His symptoms have greatly improved, and he says it's because he eats little fat, no gluten and takes a substantial supplement of vitamins and minerals. The MacDougal diet helped its creator, and he shares it in the hope that it will help others.

18. Unusual, dubious and unorthodox treatments

At this point in the book, we are fairly well informed about the treatment of multiple sclerosis. We are aware, at least, of what is taught in Medical School and what is prescribed in public health centers.

But there is also an odd array of unorthodox treatments out there, whose value is questionable. Some are too recent to have made their way into the mainstream; others have been proposed in the absence of a solid scientific base, but may suggest new therapeutical lines. These are imaginative prescriptions, not necessarily accredited ones. Perhaps one day some of these intuitive attempts will make a real contribution to the fight against multiple sclerosis. There is such a thing as a lucky guess.

AGAINST SPASTICITY AND AGAINST THE LAW

There are illegal drugs that can serve to reduce spasticity. Marijuana (or cannabis) alleviates spasticity in 97% of the patients who report using it. It also improves chronic pain, appetite, memory and mood, fatigue, vision, gait, balance, sexual alterations, and bladder or intestinal alterations. Patients with multiple sclerosis have good therapeutic reasons for smoking cannabis.[87]

Cocaine, "crack," morphine, or heroin can produce a sensation of well-being, and they may alleviate the spasticity or pain, but at the expense of very serious side effects and the problem of addiction.

A TOXIN RIGHT OUT OF A CAN

Cans of food that have spoiled contain an anaerobic microorganism, *Clostridium botulinum*. It secretes such a potent toxin that the person who ingests it dies of suffocation, because it paralyzes the respiratory muscles.

But there is a silver lining: this botulinus toxin is a powerul muscle relaxant. If we inject very tiny fractions of the toxin into one or more specific muscles, we can get them to relax for weeks or months. This method is very effective in suppressing certain abnormal movements (facial muscle spasms). It has not been approved as a treatment for multiple sclerosis, but it may solve a situation of intense local spasticity.[218]

GIVEN A MEDULLA TRANSPLANT, SHE DIES

In February of 1996, a medical researcher from Wisconsin decided to try transplanting bone marrow to treat multiple sclerosis. At the end of that year, he applied the therapy to 49-year-old Connie Lieske. She died on June 30, 1997.

OPERATING ON VERTEBRAL ARTERIES

There are private clinics that offer surgical treatment of multiple sclerosis by, according to them, improving the blood flow in the vertebral arteries. In reality, they usually perform a routine operation of supposed stenosis of the scalene muscle pass. I find the notion outrageous, expensive and useless, but there are still doctors who do it and patients who have it done.

GOD, THE ALMIGHTY APOTHECARY

Countering these risky techniques are the naturalistic doctrines, modern versions of Paracelsus:[i] *"God, the almighty apothecary, would have provided in Nature specific remedies for every disease, which the alchemist was to know and isolate."*

Treatment, then, consists of finding the plant or "natural" chemical element that is lacking in the ill person.

COBRA VENOM AT THE PHARMACY

A person is bitten by a cobra, and from the symptoms doctors deduce that his nervous system has undergone a very special type of stimulation.

Later, they do tests with the cobra venom (alone or mixed with venom from two other snake types) and appraise the results. They conclude that the venom is an immunological stimulant, rich in nerve growth factors, and that it has a certain antiviral, analgesic and anti-inflammatory capacity.

Since then, the triple snake venom has been used for multiple sclerosis, arthritis, lupus, herpes, muscular dystrophy, Parkinson's disease, myasthenia gravis and amyotrophic lateral sclerosis.[490]

There is no solid scientific data to back up these claims, and the treatment may even be dangerous, but it can be purchased in German pharmacies (Horvi MS), and some doctors in Florida continue to prescribe it (there they call it Proven).

BEES AND MULTIPLE SCLEROSIS

Nearly all of us have been stung by a bee at some time. Multiple sclerosis patients, too.

Some of them say that the sting provoked a new exacerbation of the disease, while others think that their symptoms improved afterward. The toxin of the beesting is still under study, but there are no clear findings.

YEAST IN THE VEINS

There are preparations made with three kinds of yeast that some dare to inject into their veins, even though it gives them a bit of fever.

They say it fortifies their defenses to infections and allergic reactions, and that it protects them from multiple sclerosis. No one has proven anything... yet.

MOTHERS WHO ATTACK THEIR CHILDREN

We ar not referring to the crime of Medea[ii]. All mothers attack their children while they are still in the uterus, simply because their immunological system perceives the fetus as a foreign entity.

To defend itself from the aggression, the liver of the fetus secretes a protein (alpha-fetoprotein) that disarms the maternal army.

The idea is a good one: if this fetal protein protects it from maternal lymphocytes and antibodies, it might work in patients with multiple sclerosis. Studies are underway.

PREGNANCY MAKES FOR A BETTER FUTURE

The way things change: years back, pregnant MS patients were advised to abort, and now it so happens that pregnancy is beneficial in the final analysis.

We already knew that there are fewer flare-ups during gestation and more in the puerperium (see Chapter 6), but we did not have reliable information about the long term effects.

The most thorough study yet[456] analyzes the evolution of these patients over a 25 year period. Those who did not have children were more incapacitated, and three times as many of them had a progressive form of the disease. Pregnancy may prove to be a therapeutic investment in the future.[224]

HEALTH AND YOUTH, WITH FETUSES

It is an ancient myth: the old or sick man secures health by taking it from the young, exuberant subject. Despite the ethical problems, human fetuses, or fetuses from cows, sheep or pigs, are used in some treatments.

A Swiss clinic took the time to inject a fetal extract of whatever organ was ailing the patient: fetal liver for those with cirrhosis, fetal brain matter for those with sclerosis.

The effect was contrary, producing an experimental allergic encephalitis, just like when rats are injected with myelin. Any logical mind would have foreseen it.

INJECTING ALLERGENS

When a person has asthma or an allergy to pollen, dust, or certain foods, he is treated with minimal amounts of those same substances so that the body "gets accustomed" to them. It is a de-sensitization, the aim being that the individual react less and less to whatever produces the allergy (the allergen).

Some apply these desensitizing treatments to multiple sclerosis, assuming that it is a type of allergy to environmental factors. It has not proven to be useful.

A COOL SPACE SUIT

Thermal suits --like those worn by astronauts-- to keep body temperature low have also been tried. There are complete suits, or others that just cover the trunk and head. The premise is evident: multiple sclerosis symptoms improve with cool temperatures, and get worse with the heat, which would make the damaged nerve fibers conduct impulses more slowly.

These personalized "cooling" or "microclimate" systems have been studied under a project by the Multiple Sclerosis Association of America (MSAA).[264,395] Other associations (for example, Inside MS, of the National Multiple Sclerosis Society) advertise them in their publications.

They claim that the suits improve coordination, fatigue and spasticity, and that they increase overall performance.[iii]

There are other temperature-reducing suits or vests that are less sophisticated than these "space suits," and much less expensive.

BACTERIA PROTECT US FROM VIRUSES

The enemies of my enemies are my friends. Bacteria can do us harm, but they protect us from viruses that may be more dangerous still; this might be the case with multiple sclerosis. We saw earlier that a similar disease can be produced in rats (experimental allergic encephalomyelitis).

Well, if the rats were previously infected with tuberculosis or whooping cough, they were protected from EAE, and demyelination did not occur.[292]

Some bacteria know how to "spar": they train with our lymphocytes, strengthen our antibodies and prevent the appearance of autoimmune diseases. Remember, "poor" children, in precarious sanitary conditions, have less multiple sclerosis.

TAI-CHI

Tai-chi is an ancient Chinese practice of meditated exercise. One concentrates on executing smooth motions designed to maintain the harmony between body and soul. Anyone can practice it, whatever their age and physical condition.

The exercises are safe, and can be modified to be done from a sitting positition. They can be taught at classes, or simply followed on video.

Tai-chi diminishes stress and fatigue, favors muscle relaxation and improves balance.[158] (In Chapter 18, one of our patients tells us how well she is doing since taking it up.)

GULPING DOWN VITAMINS

There is also a theory that multiple sclerosis is caused by a vitamin deficiency. Every vitamin possible, and many different minerals, are tried in every imaginable combination and dosage. But the ones taken most are vitamins A and C, which, in large doses, can be harmful.

CAREFUL WITH THE IRON

Iron is accumulated in the brains of patients with different neurological diseases, and the pattern may be characterisitc of inflammatory processes or those of another sort. o de otra índole[482].

Autopsies have revealed high concentrations of iron in the brains of subjects who had multiple sclerosis. That led to an analysis of transferrin (the protein that binds and transports iron in the blood) in live MS patients. It was found at high levels, particularly in the more incapacitated patients.[531]

BROAD-SPECTRUM ANTIBIOTICS

There is also a theory about multiple sclerosis being related to a bacterial infection. Terramycin, Tetracycline and other such antibiotics with a broad spectrum of action (effective against very different bacterial classes) have been tried.

And just in case the cause is a fungus, others treat with nystatin, a substance that is used when these organisms infect the mouth or vagina. All in vain.

GYPSY BLOOD

This idea occurred to my friend Hyde[iv] as we were gazing at the Alhambra of Granada, surrounded by gypsy women who tried to sell flowers to the tourists and read their palms. "You know, this might just be the remedy for multiple sclerosis: gypsy blood."

And then he went on to explain the astounding hypothesis: "In your book you state that MS patients have toxic substances in the blood serum that attack the myelin, and that is why the exacerbations can be treated with plamspheresis, or replacing the patient's antibodies withr ones from a donor."

There was a twinkle in his eye as he got to the point, as if it were a dark secret: "All you have to do is select the donors. If gypsies are immune to the disease, let's ask them to donate their blood. Maybe that Harvard student who is hardly able to walk would get better with two or three liters of gypsy blood."

And at once my friend changed the subject, insisting we move on to his favorite old-fasioned tavern, where he ordered a pitcher of beer and a dish of olives, and he lit up a *Camel*. We never mentioned the topic again.

ACUPUCTURE

The Chinese have been practicing it for four thousand years. Needles are inserted into different sites on the body that are believed to correspond to the functioning of certain organs.

In reality they produce a sensitve afference to diverse areas of the nervous system, and they have been shown to relaease substances such as endorphins (a kind of "natural" morphine) that serve to alleviate pains or muscle spasms. But it does not cure multiple sclerosis.

NERVE STIMULATION

It can be considered as a variation of acupuncture. Instead of inserting needles to excite the nearby nerve fibers, the nerve is stimulated directly, by placing electrodes on the skin above and applying electricity at different intensities.

No controlled studies have been published, but it is a form of interfering with the nervous system that might have future applications in this or other diseases..

MAGNETISM FOR DREAMING

With multiple sclerosis, dreaming is altered, as well as the capacity to recall dreams upon awaking.

According to some,[463] one dreams more and remembers his dreams when electromagnetic fields are applied (in addition to helping improve other symptoms of the disease). The evolution of the chronic progressive forms is even said to improve.[461,465,466].

Magnetotherapy acts more or less like repeated high-frequency stimulations of the nerve fibers that are below the field where it is applied.

THE PRESSURIZED OXYGEN FASHION

Fashions come and go in the medical world as well. Treating multiple sclerosis with hyperbaric oxygen was in vogue in the 80's.

It consisted of giving oxygen at higher than usual pressures so that it would penetrate into the bloodstream better.

It is a procedure used for some burns, for air embolisms (divers' decompression chambers) or in patients with gas gangrene (produced by germs that are killed by oxygen).

In the U.S., England, Italy and Russia, thousands of persons with multiple sclerosis used it... until six separate, controlled double-blind studies, with the help of magnetic resonance imaging, showed that there were no significant results.

SURRENDERING TO PLEASURES[v]

Pleasure and health bear a close relation, one that was upheld ages ago by Epicureans, and later negated by Stoics and Christians.

The notion is now coming to life again: in order to enjoy good health, it is necessary to enjoy some of life's pleasures.

COW HEART, PIG PANCREAS

Take a cow heart. Put it in a container with some pig pancreas extract to digest it, and add water. That is how you obtain a protein solution that is used for certain bacterial cultures.

Well some individuals found another use for it: they injected it into the veins of multiple sclerosis patients, in an attempt to cure them. Some got worse, others got a lot worse. Inexcuseable.

MULTIPURPOSE ALCOHOL

Octacosanol is a simple, long-chain alcohol, which is believed (by some) to favor the incorporation of fatty acids to myelin lipids. Not only has it been tried in treating multiple sclerosis; it has also been used for amyotrophic lateral sclerosis, (a disease that has nothing to do with MS), myesthenia gravis, muscular dystrophies, dermatomyositis, cerebral palsy and other processes.

No objective data stands in its favor.

ELECTRONIC SPINAL CORD

Electric stimulators of the spinal cord have also been developed. They are used to improve spasticity and incontinence. My colleague López del Val tells us about them in Chapter 20.

THE FIRST MILK AFTER BIRTH

The first milk that the mother gives her nursing newborn is called colostrum,[70] and it is rich in antibodies. Cow's milk has more antibodies than human milk, because the antibodies cannot permeate the placenta of the mother cow, and so they must be given to the baby calf after birth.

The colostrum of a cow can be further enriched in defenses if the animal is vaccinated against a series of viruses while pregnant. When the animal gives birth, the foremilk is extracted, frozen, and later given to multiple sclerosis patients.[vi] Studies of this treatment have been undertaken in Japan and the United States, but with deficient controls and uncertain conclusions.[490]

SPIRULINE

Spiruline is an algae. The Ucranians of the Carpathian mountain region eat quite a bit of it, and it appears that the periods of remission for the multiple sclerosis patients living in this area are more prolonged.[62]

UTOPIAS AND CHIMERAS

They are wild stabs at treating with no solid foundation. A utopia is something one can dream of or hope for, but that does not exist anywhere (*u-topos*: not in any place). Fanciful creations are called chimeras.[vii] These terms could be applied to some of the following treatments, which promise benefits that are never substantiated.

Proteolytic enzymes: a mixture of digestive enzymes (pancreatin, chymotrypsin and others) is given intravenously.

Procaine: a local anesthetic that is injected when performing local surgery, or applied in cream for sunburn. It has been used in capsule form for multiple sclerosis and to improve mental and physical functions.

Ultrasound: a diagnostic method used widely to study arteries, the abdomen, or fetal development. Some apply high frequency sounds repeatedly to the vertebral column in an attempt to improve multiple sclerosis symptoms.

REMOVAL OF THE UTERUS

Some multiple sclerosis patients have undergone a hysterectomy in order to modify their hormonal situation, and therfore their immune system as well. It entails the risks of a major surgical intervention, and serves no purpose.

THE ANTIDOTE NAMED "CHELATE"

In children's stories, when a person drinks poison, there is supposedly an antidote somewhere --that is, a substance which, if taken soon enough, can remove the toxin from the bloodstream.

In medicine there are some honest-to-goodness antidotes known as chelates. If someone has lead poisoning, his blood is full of this metal; he is given a chelate that combines with the metal and is later eliminated. And so the patient is "detoxified."

Some people are convinced that multiple sclerosis is caused by toxic substances, and they try to get rid of them by introducing chelates such as EDTA (ethylenediaminetetraacetic acid), by itself or in combination with others,[490] as in the formula marketed in Rumania under the name Rodilemid.

Not only are they expensive; they can be mortal if not administered properly.

REVITALIZING WITH RABBIT ANTIBODIES

The thymus, bone marrow, the spleen and the placenta are tissues that, in one way or another, play a role in immunological action. A Russian scientist made a mixture of all of the above, injected it into rabbits, and obtained "anti-immunological tissue antibodies."

Then he gave it to humans in small, repeated doses, and said that it stimulated their defenses.

It was claimed to be an "immunological revitalization" that has since been tried in patients with allergies or cancer, as an aphrodisiac, and to prolong life. It was also used to treat multiple sclerosis (a study was done in the late 70's). Besides being useless, it is very costly.

INJECTING YOUR OWN BACTERIA

We're talking about autogenic vaccines. In keeping with the old theory that some diseases are allergic reactions to the germs within one's own body, bacteria could be taken from the patient, cultured, and then reintroduced (injected) as vaccines. This treatment has a solid basis: bacteria or their derivatives exert an influence on the production of interferon; but since there is no way to control what is being done (the treatment has not been commercialized or regulated), it may be dangerous.[490]

PROVOKING THE ENEMY

Proneut: a combination of histamine with the measles vaccine and the vaccine for the form of influenza Europeans know as "grippe." It is a "provocation/neutralizacion" treatment with these three components that are suspected of causing multiple sclerosis.

FORTIFYING THE CONJUNTIVE TISSUE

Veterinarians use certain enzymes[viii] for chronic inflammations, in order to strengthen the animal's conjunctive tissue. Some have applied the idea to cures for old age. In a study of 20 patients with multiple scleroisis, there was talk of improvement, but the data were not presented objectively. At least there were no toxic effects.[490]

A CHEAP, OVER-THE-COUNTER LINIMENT

With a little bit of money, and without a prescription, we can purchase a liniment called dimethyl sulfoxide.

It is rapidly absorbed in the skin, and rubbing it in can alleviate cramps, muscle contractures, and pain in the joints. In animals it exerts an immunosuppressive effect, and tests are being run to see if it works in autoimmune diseases when used on the skin (as a liniment), orally, or by injection. It has not been tested in humans, and we have no idea of the risks involved.

PIG BRAIN GRAFTS

Only authentic despair or twisted information can explain something like this. Thirty-eight Germans with multiple sclerosis paid to have a piece of pig brain implanted in their abdomens. A graft of a foreign animal part has unforseeable immunological consequences.

Two suffered serious complications, and one patient died. Another transplant resulted in a case of polyradiculoneuropathy, and it was shown that the patient was sensitized to cerebral gangliosides.[260]

OZONE AS A CURE-ALL

So many miracles at once are hard to believe. In Greece they use Alfasal a product containing ozone, obtained by electrolyzing a saline solution.

It is given orally or injected to treat multiple sclerosis, cancer and 50 other diseases. Too good to be true.

SOME ALTERNATIVES WORK

Some alternative treatments may work, others do not, and others can do much more harm than good.

A study evaluated their overall usefulness[130] and they were shown to be effective: patients who, in addition to orthodox medical treatment, followed one or more alternative therapies had less severe symptoms, better functional capacity and a higher degree of quality in daily living.

UNMASKING THE SWINDLERS

There are costly alternative treatments that are ineffective and even dangerous. It is very easy to raise false hopes among persons with chronic health problems, and some take advantage of the situation. The National Society of Multiple Sclerosis offers some tips for spotting the swindlers.

We should suspect fraud when: a "cure" for multiple sclerosis is advertised; treatment must be paid for in advance; it is a secret formula; the "healer" does not want the patient to consult her regular doctor; it is marketed by telephone; or the testimony of "satisfied customers" is given with little or no identification.[158]

THE LYMPHOCYTES OF HERNÁN CORTÉS

Hernán Cortés was a man with a great deal of powerful lymphocytes in his system, just like his soldiers. A handful of Spanish explorers were able to conquer the Aztec empire thanks to their immunity to the diseases they transmitted.

"The Spanish conquerers who invaded the "New World" were immunological supermen. They came from a natural, darwinian selection, because the Spanish ports on the Mediterranean and the Atlantic coasts harbored people and germs from Europe, Africa, Asia and America, and childhood infections were devastating. The Spanish sailors were survivors of these diseases, having developed very powerful immune systems. That was what gave them the advantage over the native Americans, who were immunologically defenseless."

This paragraph was taken from a book on the history of Medicine[408] given to me by my friend Hyde (the heterodox neurologist I spoke of earlier) the last time he came to visit me in Granada. He read this excerpt to me aloud and related it to the failures of the immune system seen in multiple sclerosis.

Then he made up a Scandinavian tale that ends in Africa, which I will now tell the rest of you.

SIGRID GOES TO MADAGASGAR

Sigrid was born in Stockholm, and was genetically predisposed to suffering from multiple sclerosis, as it affected her older sister and her grandmother.

Her father was a doctor and he decided to get a new outlook on life. He signed up to do medical work with a non-governmental organization, and the whole family moved to Madagascar.

Sigrid was just a year old when they arrived in the village. There she came down with many childhood infections that had been erradicated in Sweden.

Her new home was not as clean as the immaculate apartment back in Stockholm. And the food she ate did not have the same hygienic and quality controls. At an early age she was climbing trees and venturing into the jungle; she often got cuts and scrapes that were not always disinfected.

Throughout her childhood, her leukocytes and antibodies had been reinforced by dealing with situations she never would have encountered in her country of origin. Her immune system had been through intensive training at an early age, and Sigrid survived and will never have multiple sclerosis.

19. The patients speak

We doctors see them as patients, but they don't think of themselves in those terms. It has taken some time for the multiple sclerosis patient to learn the name of his disease. This man or woman began losing their eyesight or noticing several annoying problems, and finally went to the specialist for confirmation of the diagnosis made by the family doctor.

THE INTRUDER

And now they feel as if an intruder had burst in on their lives. "Everything was going so well with my work, my family, my friends," they say to themselves. "Just what is this sickness that I've got to deal with now? How long will it last? Maybe after a few months of treatment I'll be cured." But the truth is, the intruder does not leave. The disease creeps forward, into more areas of the person's life, as he or she tries to hide it from coworkers and acquaintances.

FROM *KIRIELEISÓN* TO THE CRY OF ORESTES

Resignation or desperation in the face of the disease. The patient may affront the cruel diagnosis with one or the other extreme. Some chant the **kirieleisón**[i] (*"Lord have pity on me"*) and feel sorry for themselves. Others will not accept the blow of misfortune and they curse fate; it is like the desperate cry of Orestes when he rebels at the divine punishment imposed upon him. *"God, if you exist, what do you* *do with your time?"*   Patients may blame "the gods" who decide human destiny for this disgrace. "Why me?" they say. "Is there no divine justice?" As we said, these attitudes represent the two extremes of a wide range of possible reactions.

FACING THE MUSIC

The time comes when everyone knows that their friend or colleague has multiple sclerosis. And they will begin to give him advice, some to cheer him up, others to let him know –intentionally or unintentionally— how terribly that same disease has affected so-and-so. Every once in a while the papers carry an news item about MS that the patient will read eagerly, but may not understand. There might also be an advertisement or sensationalistic article about a new treatment that will send the patient running to the phone to ask his doctor if it might help.

Other times despair kicks in. "I'm not getting any better, only worse, and everyone notices the way I walk. I can't bear to go out with my old friends, they look at me as if I were a stranger to them." And then there are periods when the patient is in higher spirits. "That last treatment really seems to have helped; I haven't had a flare-up for over a year. Could it be that I´m cured?"

DARE TO KNOW

Should the patient know as much as possible about his disease? With some exceptions (hypochondriacs), being knowledgeable about one's condition is not bad, it is beneficial. Most multiple sclerosis patients are young, intelligent people, and they can get much more out of life if they know just how the lesions are affecting their brain functions, how medications work, and the possible complications that may present themselves.

There are some excellent guides that will inform the patient about this disease, in Spanish or English. We will always insist that the patient, when in doubt, consult either his general physician or the neurologist. But we must encourage him not to be afraid of knowledge about his condition. *"Sapere aude"* ("Dare to know") was the advice of Horace.

HOW DO THE PATIENTS REALLY FEEL?

Even though we have spent many years treating cases of multiple sclerosis, we have not really experienced the personal perception of the disease. The interiorization of this disorder cannot be learned from journals or medical meetings; only a sensitive, communicative patient can help us comprehend it. With great respect for the afflictions of others, and unwilling to silence them prudishly, I transcribe below the tales of some patients that will help us get to know the disease from the inside out.

BATTLES WITH MY BLADDER
Gmarc[ii]

Tell me if these scenarios sound familiar to you. You are driving your car to work and feel the urge to urinate immediately. You speed up, run through a couple of stop signs, and meanwhile you've got your legs crossed and pressed together as tightly as possible. You park, your legs still pressed tight, and stumble into the bathroom feeling like you are about to burst. You loosen your clothing and throw it on the floor and... NOTHING. The urgent need to urinate has disappeared.

Or... You have gone to the bathroom to urinate. Your friends are waiting for you at the door to go see a show together, and it's getting very late. You just closed the bathroom door behind you when you feel the need to go again, and you walk back in. Finally you are ready to leave, and you are walking to the show while apologizing for the delay, and all of a sudden you feel the urgent need for a bathroom once more. "See you later, guys; I'll look for you inside the theater."

Or... It is time to go to bed, and you are very tired. You didn't sleep well the night before, and that affected your gait all day long. So tonight you are going to get a good night's sleep. After brushing your teeth, you use the toilet and crawl under the covers. You can guess the next part: it is three o'clock in the morning and you have to get up to urinate. Getting back to sleep afterwards is not so easy, and you know that in the morning you will be in poor shape again, just like the day before.

MARITA DISCOVERED TAI-CHI

Marita was a patient of mine. For some reason, we lost track of each other over the years. It was fifteen years later that I ran into her again, and she was doing very well. She told me her story:

All I know is that twenty years ago —I'm 48 now— doctors told me to buy a wheelchair. But a year and a half ago I threw out my crutches and bought myself a light cane instead. And if this keeps up, I'll get something sportier than a cane.

I discovered Tai Chi Chuan by chance, thanks to the recommendation of a nurse friend of mine who thought it might help me. I had to do the movements while seated at the first classes because my legs wouldn't respond, and my teacher was watching to make sure I didn't fall out of my chair.

I began the classes with a group of beginners, which was great, and now, if you don't mind my saying so, I'm the best in my group, and sometimes my classmates are told to watch me and follow my example. We began with the self-massages, concentration, and energy-channeling that the Chinese call "Chi Kung."

The exercises, or "forms" of Tai Chi are not at all easy, and they take a lot of concentration and dedication. It's something you have absolutely got to practice every day, if only for a little while. But it's easy, too, because you can see the results. Besides, knowing that I am taking the reins in solving my "problem" is a very reassuring feeling. Our group meets with the teacher and some other pupils of hers three or four times a year to get away from the city and practice Tai Chi together in different places, learning things from one another.

I am convinced that my body is fighting multiple sclerosis. I might never dance the cancan again, but I'm sure I will live a practically normal life. And I do not plan on investing in a wheelchair.

MATERNAL INTUITION

Mothers speak right up: "I think my daughter's (or son's) disease comes from this or that..." Women's intuition --especially from a mother-- is a road to knowledge that should not be underestimated in unraveling secrets.

A suggestion, whether scientifically founded or not, might point us in the right direction as we search for the key to multiple sclerosis. So let's listen:

GRANDFATHER'S BEEHIVE

"When she was nine, they went to see the beehives that her grandfather kept, and she got a lot of beestings. Couldn't it be from that?"

Well we can't say for certain. But that mother with no medical background had the same idea as some researchers who are now working on an important project. ¿???? //un importante proyecto de la

GROWTH INJECTIONS

"I feel sure that it's from those damned injections that she got to spur her growth."

That is the opinion of the mother of a tiny girl who was taken to the endocrinologist and given injections of somatotropin (growth hormone).

One year later she developed a rare form of multiple sclerosis: a ten year girl, with primary chronic evolution.

20. The doctors speak

Each of them has something to do (much to do) with multiple sclerosis. Some have chosen to dedicate themselves to basic research, some to teaching, and others (the majority) to clinical work in different specialties: Neurology, Ophthalmology, or Psychiatry. Each one responds to a question from his personal viewpoint, with the authority conferred by knowledge and first-hand experience.

WHAT IS MYELIN?

José Mª Peinado Herreros[i].

In the nervous system, the classic distinction is between white matter (which contains the "myelinated" axons and glial cells), and the gray matter (where nerve cells and their dendritic branches predominate).

Myelin is the principal component of the so-called myelin sheaths. In the Central Nervous System, the sheaths are made by the oligodendrocytes, and in the Peripheral Nervous System they are formed by Schwann cells. The sheaths are wound around the neural axons, modifying to a great extent the nerve-signal conductivity of the membrane of these axons.

These coverings surround the axon, like the plastic that covers electrical wires, but with an important difference: the covering is not continuous, but periodically interrupted, leaving myelin-free segments of the axons that are known as Ranvier nodes. Between one node and the next, a Schwann cell or an oligodendroglia forms a myelin sheath. The myelin sheaths increase the thickness of the axon membrane substantially, thereby increasing its resistance to the electrical current. This means that the nerve signal is transmitted via the low-resistance, myelin-free intervals, the Ranvier nodes, traveling from axon to axon in a jumping fashion, much quicker and more effectively than would be the case in demyelinated axons.

Myelination is a fundamental factor in increasing the velocity of nerve fiber conductivity. The other evolutive strategy used by nature to enhance conductivity is increasing the axon diameter. A myelinated axon takes up $1/100^{th}$ of the volume of a non-mylinated axon transmitting signals at the same speed. Considering the number of axons that are in the average human brain, its volume would have to increase by more than 10 times in order for the demyelinated axons to conduct signals at the same rate as myelinated ones.

The myelin sheaths are formed by the addition of oligodendrocyte membranes or Schwann cell membranes without cytoplasm, as if the membrane of the axon surrounded itself with many other membrane layers.

But, what is a cell membrane? A cell membrane is made up of a double layer of lipids, in which proteins are integrated. The molecular composition of these myelin sheaths is 30% protein and 70% lipid, of which nearly 25% are cerebrosides, and another 25% cholesterol. The rest are other lipids, some of them of a polar nature, among which the so-called sphingomyelins constitute no more than 10%.

THE OPHTHALMOLOGIST SEES AN OPTIC NEURITIS

Daniel Serrano[ii]

When a patient discovers that his visual acuity has suddenly diminished, he always attributes it to the peripheral receptor organ (the eyeball), and goes to the ophthalmologist. The patient does not know that the visual organ comprises not only the eye (the receptor) but also the optic pathway (which relays the information) and the occipital cortex (which interprets what is seen). The ophthalmologist is in charge of the eyeball, while the neurologist takes care of the rest of the visual system.

When an ophthalmologist encounters an optic neuritis, the first problem is in the differential diagnosis with ischemic optic neuropathy. But even though the consequences for vision would be similar, the prognosis is different for the two diseases. For this reason, and because a neuritis is the expression of a more important generalized process (demyelination), these cases must be referred to the neurologist (in addition to correcting the risk factors of local ischemic processes, most notably high blood pressure.)

The ophthalmologist fulfills the fundamental service of indicating to the neurologist the evolution of the neuritic process (determination and evaluation of the visual field, visual acuity and pupillary reflexes). Through the findings of the ophthamological examination, the neurologist can modulate the therapy to be followed in each particular case.

ARE MY URINARY PROBLEMS BECAUSE OF MS?

Juan Andrés Burguera Hernández[iii]

Between 60 and 80% of the patients with multiple sclerosis present urinary disorders at some point in their evolution. In one in ten patients, they are present at the time of the first exacerbation, and in one in one hundred, isolated urinary symptoms constitute the first flare-up. The progression of the neurological affectation is associated with a greater deterioration of the bladder-sphincter function.

This is due to the location and the extension of the demyelinating lesions, which interrupt the connections of the brain and the spinal cord with the bladder that regulate its voluntary control, thus disturbing the functions of the storing and emptying of urine. The symptoms may be irritable or obstructive. The most frequent irritable symptoms are urgency, increased urine, urinary incontinence, bladder or urethral discomfort, or the constant desire to urinate. The obstructive symptoms are difficulty in initiating miction, weak flow, postmictional leakage, interruption of flow, urinary retention, and nicturia. In 18 to 52 (%?)of patients there is a combination of both symptomologies.

These urinary disorders may condition the long term prognosis of the disease due to the appearance of infectious complications or kidney trouble. In addition, they significantly affect the quality of life and the self-esteem of these patients, by limiting them in their daily work and social activities. There are adequate means for correctly diagnosing these disorders, which are nearly always treatable, and can sometimes be cured.

IS LUMBAR PUNCTURE NECESSARY?

Miguel Guerrero Fernández[iv]

Yes, it is necessary, because it permits us to analyze the cerebrospinal fluid, the only way of knowing what is happening within the central nervous system (brain and spinal cord). When we think a person has anemia, we request a hemogram; when a person with bronchitis is in the Emergency room with serious trouble breathing, we prick his radial artery to measure the oxygen it carries, and when a gastric ulcer is suspected, an endoscopy is done (those well-known "rubber tubes") to confirm the diagnosis. Either one of the latter two tests is more bothersome for the patient than a lumbar puncture to examine the cerebrospinal fluid (CSF).

It is very important to diagnose multiple sclerosis and offer a prognosis of the form in which the patient will evolve. The initial symptoms may not be typical, or the magnetic resonance imaging may show normal (in the case of spinal cord lesions), or else the evoked potentials might show no alterations. In these cases the CSF study is crucial, as it reveals the alterations of the lymphocytes or immunoglobulins, contributes to research, and, above all, serves to confirm diagnosis.

The lumbar puncture requested and performed by an expert neurologist entails practically no risk, and is not painful, especially when local anesthesia is given (some patients say they "never even noticed the puncture" when it is over). Nonetheless, why do patients dread it so? It is probably associated with diseases that were formerly very serious or invalidating (meningitis, syphilis), and years ago it was done without the previous control of a scanner, for which reason, in cases of tumors, there was a risk of piercing. At present, with the studies of cerebral visualization we now have, that complication is highly improbable. Some patients, after the puncture, present a headache, which characteristically appears when they stand up or have been seated for a while, and goes away completly when they lie down and rest, drinking plenty of liquids for a few days. This type of headache, called a "spinal headache" ¿?? CSF hypotension headache ¿?, when it occurs, is totally benign and leaves no sequelae. So let us destroy the black legend of the lumbar puncture: it is not so dangerous, nor as bothersome as other tests that are done routinely in our hospitals.

IS THERE A TYPICAL MS PERSONALITY?

José Luis Jiménez Bullejos[v]

Multiple sclerosis patients relate with each other in a unique way when they coincide at the psychiatrist's office. It's as if there were a disassociation between what the verbal and emotional realms, between what is expressed and what is felt. They are close to what Liberman calls personalities that resort to a conversive (or infantile) technique in relating to each other. // de relación conversiva (o infantil).

For these patients, the somtic syndrome constitutes, at the same time, pessimism, feeling, and action. They know a lot about "their disease," diagnosis, flare-ups, pills and injections... but little or nothing about themselves; nor do they seem very concerned about it. They produce a particular kind of countertransference at the Psychiatrist's, as if the emotional aspects of discourse had no meaning, so that a "de-affective" encounter with the other is produced; in psychological terms, it results in a "book dialogue."

At some point in time, the multiple sclerosis patient presents symptoms of depression. It is then, we believe, that we can take advantage of the circumstance to try to get them to connect more with their internal world, to be a bit more introspective. If we succeed, they will get to know themselves better; and even though at first the process may not be enjoyable, it will be in their benefit to experience it in a more analytical and enriching manner.

IS ELECTRICAL STIMULATION OF THE MEDULLA OF ANY USE?

Luis Javier López del Val[vi]

It is evident that epidural electrical stimulation does not cure the disease, but it is doubtless one more therapeutic alternative we can use in our repertory of symptomatic treatment. Epidural electrical neurostimulation achieves important improvement in the spasticity of lower members, secondarily improving the patient's gait and allowing him greater mobility; at the same time, it improves bladder hyperreflexia, increasing residual capacity, and decreasing the uninhibited contractions that cause incontinence.

The technique is relatively simple: with the patient awake, lying face down, we perform a lumbar puncture to introduce, under radioscopic control, a wire that has four poles at its end (tetrapolar) or eight poles (octopolar) into the epidural space, approximately at the level of the D9-D10 (above the dorsal mictional circuit). The distal end of the wire is tunneled under the skin to the lumbar fossa or to the iliac fossa, where it is connected to an electric generator. Usually this is done in two sessions, leaving the patient with an external stimulation for a few days to evaluate the response, and the second time the tunneling is carried out with the connection to the final generator.

It is important to underline the absence of complications attibutable to the neurostimulator in the 40-some patients with multiple sclerosis that we have treated. Of course, all our patients have gotten worse over time, as the evolution of the disease does not vary with stimultion; but the quality of the improvement obtained makes this an excellent option to be considered in the symptomatic treatment of complications, above all in patients who show an acceptable degree of clinical stability.

HOW IS MULTIPLE SCLEROSIS TAUGHT AT MEDICAL SCHOOL?

Alfonso Castro García[vii]

The teaching of Neurology at Medical School always was and is still in the hands of Internists, and therefore multiple sclerosis, in most of the universities of Spain, is still explained by these professors. Suffice it to say that at present there are very few professors of Neurology who impart this discipline. In fact, there are only six Chairs in Neurology in this country, and a few more tenured professors of Neurology.

Obviously then the chapter on demyelinating diseases is being explained, in most cases, by professors who do not habitually treat or have a first-hand knowledge of multiplie sclerosis patients.

21. The future can only be brighter

Technology and science are advancing so rapidly that the future can only be brighter for those who depend on new medical breakthroughs. In the past few years some effective treatments for multiple sclerosis have become widespread: interferons, copolymers, growth factors, etc. It is now a "treatable" disease; and most importantly, new doors have opened, generating optimism about further progress, perhaps right around the corner.[341]

THERE WILL BE A CURE, AND WE'LL ALL KNOW

The patient should keep informed about scientific progress and, if he so wishes, about alternative treatments as well. But he should not be obsessed with seeking more sources of information, because when an effective treatment for multiple sclerosis comes out, the social repercussions will be enormous.

There will be a cure, and we are certain to hear about it. The mass media –newspapers, the radio, TV, Internet—will all announce the news immediately, all over the world. May that day come soon.

AND OTHERS WILL REAP THE BENEFITS, TOO

So much time and money is being invested in research about multiple sclerosis that patients with other autoimmune diseases can find reason to be hopeful as well. The discoveries surrounding the pathogeny and treatment of multiple sclerosis are followed eagerly by persons with rheumatoid arthritis, diabetes and other diseases.[433]

HOW DOES SCIENCE MOVE FORWARD?

At the moment, MS researchers are working on a number of assumptions//premises: damage to the myelin, auto-immunity, chromosome 6, interferon... At some point one of these scientific foundations might offer a new interpretation, or a new aspect might arise to explain matters that were incomprehensible until now, thereby opening up new roads to treatment. It will be a "scientific revolution" in the sense used by Kuhn:[266]

"In order to discover something, we must first perceive an anomaly; then, see if our concepts, and the procedures based on them, can solve the enigma; and finally, if they cannot, then we must look for others that might.".

This change represents the scientific revolution, and it is the nucleus of a theory about scientific progress.

HOPING WHILE WAITING

We have come to the end of a book that should not end. Every day there are new data, new drugs, new expectations in the face of this disease. One day we will learn the truth about multiple sclerosis, and it may be very surprising.

In future editions of this book, it is hoped, we will offer summaries and updates of all the biomedical advancements that have taken place in the interim. And I would like to add more opinions and input from patients and their family members. I have learned a lot from them, directly or over Internet. Any contribution may prove useful; a disease that has this many mysteries for us to solve can be approached from unsuspected directions.

Imagination. We need to use our imagination in fighting multiple sclerosis. I hereby request the reader's collaboration: you may send to the electronic address below any bit of information or hypothesis about the disease that you find relevant. Or, if you have the urge, suggestions for improving this book in future editions. Thank you..

info@neuroconsulta.com
www.gonzalezmaldonado.com

....

References and Footnotes

REFERENCES

1.   Abramsky O, Lehmann D, Karussis D. Immunomodulation with linomide: possible novel therapy for multiple sclerosis. Mult Scler 1996; 2: 206-210.

2.   Achiron A, Gabbay U, Gilad R, Hassin Baer S, Barak Y, Gornish M, Elizur A, Goldhammer Y, Sarova Pinhas I. Intravenous immunoglobulin treatment in multiple sclerosis. Effect on relapses. Neurology 1998; 50: 398-402

3.   Adams RD, Victor M. Principles of Neurology. McGraw-Hill, New York 1995.

4.   Agranoff BW, Goldberg D. Diet and the geographical distribution of multiple sclerosis. Lancet 1974; ii: 1061-1066.

5.   Alaev BA, Aslanov AM. [Familial cases of multiple sclerosis when siblings reside in different climato-geographical zones]. O semeinykh sluchaiakh rasseiannogo skleroza pri prozhivanii sibsov v raznykh klimatogeograficheskikh regionakh. Zh Nevropatol Psikhiatr Im S S Korsakova 1987; 87:370-373.

6.   Albiac G. Mentes sifilíticas. El Mundo, 20/10/97.

7.   Al-Din AS. Multiple sclerosis in Kuwait: clinical and epidemiological study. J Neurol Neurosurg Psychiatry 1986; 49:928-931.

8.   Al-Din AS, Khogali M, Poser CM, al-Nassar KE, Shakir R, Hussain J, Behbahani K, Chadha G. Epidemiology of multiple sclerosis in Arabs in Kuwait: a comparative study between Kuwaitis and Palestinians. J Neurol Sci 1990; 100: 137-141.

9.   Al-Din ASN, Kurdi A, Mubaidin A, El-Khateeb M. Epidemiology of multiple sclerosis in Arabs in Jordan: a comparative study between Jordanians and Palestinians. J Neurol Sci 1996; 135:162-167.

10.   Allen K, Blascovich J. The value of service dogs for people with severe ambulatory disabilities. A randomized controlled trial. JAMA 1996; 275: 1001-1006.

11.   Alter N, Yamoor M, Harshe M. Multiple sclerosis and nutrition. Arch Neurol 1974; 31: 267-272.

12.   Amato MP, Ponziani G, Pracucci G, Bracco L, Siracusa G, Amaducci L. Cognitive impairment in early-onset multiple sclerosis: pattern, predictors, and impact on everyday life in a 4-year follow-up. Arch Neurol 1995; 52:168-172.

13. Amer Ferrer G, Isla A, Díez Tejedor E, Roda JM, Hernández Pérez MA, Barreiro Tella P. Lesiones de esclerosis multiple que simulan un proceso expansivo en la TC. Neurología 1990; 5:208-211.

14. Andersen O, Lycke J, Tollesson PO, Svenningsson A, Runmarker B, Linde AS, Astrom M, Gjorstrup P, Ekholm S. Linomide reduces the rate of active lesions in relapsing-remitting multiple sclerosis. Neurology 1996; 47: 895-900.

15. Anderson DW, Ellenberg JH, Leventhal CM, Reingold SC, Rodriguez M, Silberberg DH. Revised estimate of the prevalence of multiple sclerosis in the United States. Ann Neurol 1992; 31:333-336.

16. Anton Aranda E, Martinez-Lage JM, Maravi Petri E, Gallego Cullere J, de Castro P, Villanueva Eusa JA. Epidemiologia y aspectos clínico-evolutivos de la esclerosis multiple en Navarra. Neurologia 1991; 6: 160-169.

17. Antonio Enrique. Retablo de luna. Antonio Ubago Ed, Granada 1980.

18. Aristóteles. La política (h. 344 aC). Editora Nacional, Madrid 1977.

19. Aromatico A. Alquimia, el secreto entre la ciencia y la filosofía. Ediciones B.S.A, Barcelona 1997.

20. Asimov I. Palabras en el mapa. Ediciones del Prado, Madrid 1994.

21. Auer RN, Rowlands CG, Perry SF, Remmers JE. Multiple sclerosis with medullary plaques and fatal sleep apnea (Ondine's curse). Clin Neuropathol 1996; 15:101-105.

22. Azzimondi G, Stracciari A, Rinaldi R, D'Alessandro R, Pazzaglia P. Multiple sclerosis with very late onset: report of six cases and review of the literature. Eur Neurol 1994; 34:332-336.

23. Bakke A, Myhr KM, Gronning M, Nyland H. Bladder, bowel and sexual dysfunction in patients with multiple sclerosis- a cohort study. Scand J Urol Nephrol 1996 (suppl); 179; 61-66.

24. Bansil S, Singhal BS, Ahuja GK, Ladiwala U, Behari M, Friede R, Cook SD. Comparison between multiple sclerosis in India and the United States: a case-control study. Neurology 1996; 46:385-387.

25. Barak Y, Achiron A, Elizur A, Gabbay U, Noy S, Sarova-Pinhas I. Sexual dysfunction in relapsing-remitting multiple sclerosis: magnetic resonance imaging, clinical, and psychological correlates. J Psychiatry Neurosci 1996; 21:255-258.

26. Barker R, Larner A. ubstance P and multiple sclerosis. Med Hypotheses 1992; 37:40-43.
27. Barkhof F, Valk J, Hommes OR et al. Gadopentetate dimeglumine enhancement of multiple sclerosis lesions on long TR spin-echo images at 0.6 T. Am J Neuroradiol 1992; 13: 1257-1259.

28. Barraquer i Bordás Ll. Prólogo. Esclerosis múltiple, una aproximación multidisciplinaria. Fernández Fernández O (ed). Arké 144 SL, Madrid 1994 (*passim*).

29. Barraquer i Bordás Ll. Sobre las formas extremadamente benignas de la esclerosis múltiple. Noticias EM 1996; 45:4-5.

30. Barroche G, Perrier P, Raffoux C, Gehin P, Streiff F, Weber M. HLA et scleroses en plaques familiales. Rev Neurol (Paris) 1986; 142:738-745.

31. Bates D. Lipids and multiple sclerosis. Biochem Soc Trans 1989; 17: 289-291.

32. Bates D. Dietary lipids and multiple sclerosis. Uppsala J Med Sci 1990; 48 (suppl): 173-187.

33. Beatty WW. Alteraciones cognos-citivas y emocionales en la esclerosis múltiple. En: Brumbarck RA (ed). Neurología conductual. Clínicas Neurológicas de Norteamérica, 1/1993. Traducción española. Nueva Editorial Interamericana, México DF 1993.

34. Beatty WW, Goodkin DE, Beatty PA et al. Frontal lobe sysfunction and memory impairment in patients with chronic progrssive multiple sclerosis. Brain Cogn 1989; 11: 73.

35. Beatty WW, Goodkin DE, Monson N et al. Anterograde and retrograde amnesia in patients with chronic progressive multiple sclerosis. Arch Neurol 1988; 45: 611.

36. Beatty WW, Goodkin DE, Monson N et al. Cognitive disturbances in patients with relapsing remitting multiple sclerosis. Arch Neurol 1989; 46: 1113.

37. Bebo BF Jr, Vandenbark AA, Offner H. Male SJL mice do not relapse after induction of EAE with PLP 139-151. J Neurosci Res 1996; 45: 680-689.

38. Beck RW, Cleary PA, Trobe JD et al. The effect of corticosteroids for acute optic neuritis on the subsequent development of multiple sclerosis. New Engl J Med 1993; 329: 1764-1769.

39. Becker CC, Gidal BE, Flemming JO. Immunotherapy in multiple sclerosis, part 1. Am J Healt-Syst Pharm 1995; 52:1985-2000.

40. Becker CC, Gidal BE, Flemming JO. Immunotherapy in multiple sclerosis, part 2. Am J Healt-Syst Pharm 1995; 52:2105-2120.

41. Bécquer GA. Rimas (1858-1868). Rimas y otros poemas. Orbis, Barcelona 1997.

42. Beebe G, Kurtzke JF, Kurland LT , Auth TL, Nazler B. Studies on the natural history of multiple sclerosis. Neurology 1967; 17: 2-17.

43. Ben-Shlomo Y, Davey Smith G. Dietary fat and multiple sclerosis. Int MSJ 1994; 1: 61-67.

44. Ben-Shlomo Y, Davey Smith G. Breast feeding and multiple sclerosis. Br Med J 1994; 309: 342.

45. Ben-Shlomo Y, Davey Smith G, Marmor MG. Dietary fat in the epidemiology of multiple sclerosis: has the situation been adequately assessed? Neuroepidemiology 1992; 11: 214-225.

46. Benz C. Coping with multiple sclerosis. A practical guide toliving with the symptoms and understanding the treatments. Vermilion, London 1993.

47. Bernardi S, Buttinelli C, Grasso MG, Millefiorini E, Pace A, Prencipe M, Fieschi C. Evolution and severity markers in 233 MS patients. Riv Neurol 1987; 57:197-200.

48. Bernardin L, Rao SM, Luchetta TL et al. A prospective, long-term, longitudinal study of cognitive dysfunction in multiple sclerosis. J Clin Exp Neuropsychol 1993; 15: 17.

49. Berr C, Puel J, Clanet M et al. Risk factors in multiple sclerosis: a population-based case-control study in Hautes-Pyrenées, France. Acta Neurol Scand 1989; 80: 46-50.

50. Berr C, Puel J, Clanet M, Ruidavets JB, Mas JL, Alperovitch A. Risk factors in multiple sclerosis: a population-based case-control study in Hautes-Pyrenees, France. Acta Neurol Scand 1989; 80:46-50.

51. Berrios GE, Quemada JI. Depressive illness in multiple sclerosis. Clinical and theoretical aspects of the association. Br J Psychiatry 1990; 156:10-16.

52. Bever CT Jr, Panitch HS, Levy HB, McFarlin DE, Johnson KP. Gamma-interferon induction in patients with chronic progressive MS. Neurology 1991; 41: 1124-1127.

53. Bierce A. Diccionario del diablo (1911). M.E. Editores, Madrid 1997.

54. Billiard M. Narcolepsie. Rev Prat 1996; 46:2428-2434.

55. Blanco ML. Comentarios al II Congreso Internacional de Barcelona sobre Dieta mediterránea, marzo 1998. Salud (suplemento), Diario "El Mundo", 12/03/98.

56. Borges JL. El jardín de senderos que se bifurcan (1941). Obras completas. Emecé, Buenos Aires 1974.

57. Bourneville DM, Guérard I. De la sclérose en plaques disseminées. A. Delahaye, Paris 1869.

58. Brod SA, Burns DK. Suppresion of relapsing experimental autoimmune encephalomyelitis in the SJL/J mouse by oral administration of type I interferons. Neurology 1994; 44:1144-1148.

59. Broman T. Management of patients with multiple sclerosis. En: Vinken PJ, Bruyn GW (eds). Multiple sclerosis and other demyelinating diseases, pp 408-425. North-Holland Publishing Co, Amsterdam 1970.

60. Bronnum-Hansen H, Koch-Henriksen NJ, Hyllested K. [Survival in disseminated sclerosis in Denmark. A nation-wide study of the period 1948-1986]. Overlevelsen ved dissemineret sklerose i Danmark. En landsdoekkende undersogelse for perioden 1948-1986. Ugeskr Laeger 1995; 157:7131-7135.

61. Brosseau L, Philippe P, Methot G, Duquette P, Haraoui B. Drug abuse as a risk factor of multiple sclerosis: case-control analysis and a study of heterogeneity. Neuroepidemiology 1993; 12:6-14.

62. Buletsa BA, Ihnatovych II, Lupych PP, Pulyk OR. [The prevalence, structure and clinical problems of multiple sclerosis in the Transcarpathian area based on epidemiological study data]. Poshyrennia, struktura i deiaki pytannia kliniky mnozhynnoho sklerozu v Zakarpatti, za danymy epidemiolohichnoho doslid-zhennia. Lik Sprava 1996; 12: 163-165.

63. Burguera Hernandez JA, Arlandis Guzman S, Sanz Chinesta S, Martinez Agullo E. Alteraciones urinarias y sexuales en la esclerosis multiple. Neurología 1998; 13: 7-12

64. Burnfield A. The psychosocial impact of multiple sclerosis. Int MSJ 1995; 2:33-35.

65. Byron GG (Lord). Diario de Cefalonia. Ediciones Júcar, Madrid 1975.

66. Caine ED, Bamford KA, Schiffer RB et al. A controlled neurpsichological comparison of Huntington's disease and multiple sclerosis. Arch Neurol 1986; 43: 249.

67. Canavero S, Bonicalzi V, Massa-Micon B. Central neurogenic pruritus: a literature review. Acta Neurol Belg 1997; 97: 244-247

68. Canavero S, Pagni CA, Duca S, Bradac GB. Spinal intramedullary cavernous angiomas: a literature meta-analysis. Surg Neurol 1994; 41:381-388.

69. Carswell R. Pathological Anatomy: illustrations on elementary forms of disease. Longman, London 1838. (Citado por Kesselring 1997.)

70. Casares J. Diccionario ideológico de la lengua española. Editorial Gustavo Gili, Barcelona 1975.

71. Casetta I, Granieri E, Malagu S, Tola MR, Paolino E, Caniatti LM, Govoni V, Monetti VC, Fainardi E. Environmental risk factors and multiple sclerosis: a community-based, case-control study in the province of Ferrara, Italy. Neuroepidemiology 1994; 13:120-128.

72. Caviglia G, Crisi A, Azzoni A, Mazza S, Pinkus L. The mechanisms of repression and isolation in multiple sclerosis as regulators of personality system: a clinical study. Schweiz Arch Neurol Psychiatr 1990; 141:209-215.

73. Cendrowski W, Wender M, Dominik W et al. Epidemiological study of multiple sclerosis in western Poland. Eur Neurol 1969; 2: 90-108.

74. Cervantes Saavedra M. El ingenioso hidalgo Don Quijote de la Mancha (1615). Obras completas. Aguilar, Madrid 1975.

75. Charcot JM. Lessons sur les Maladies du Systeme Nerveux faites à la Salpêtrière (1872-1873). A. Delahaye, Paris.

76. Charcot JM. Lectures on the diseases of the nervous system. Delivered at la Salpêtrière. New Sydenham Society, London 1877.

77. Chrousos GP, Wilder RL, Gold PW. The stress response and the regulation of inflammatory disease. Ann Intern Med 1992; 117: 854-866.

78. Clarke T, Wadhwa U, Leroi I. Psychotic depression. An atypical initial presentation of multiple sclerosis. Psychosomatics 1998; 39: 72-75

79. Clavell J. Shogun. Plaza y Janés, Barcelona 1995.

80. Clayton Love WM, Reynolds M, Cashel A, Callaghan N. Fatty acid patterns of serum lipids in multiple sclerosis and other diseases. Biochem Soc Trans 1973; 1: 141-143.

81. Comi G, Filippi M, Martinelli V et al. Brain magnetic resonance imaging correlates of cognitive impairment in multiple sclerosis. J Neurol Sci 1993; 115(suppl): 66-73.

82. Compston A. Remyelination of the central nervous system. Mult Scler 1996; 1: 388-392.

83. Compston DAS. The 150th anniversary of the first depiction of the lesions of multiple sclerosis. J Neurol Neurosurg Psychiatry 1988; 51:1249-1252.

84. Compston DAS. The dissemination of multiple sclerosis. J Roy Coll Phys 1990; 24: 207-218.

85. Compston DAS. Limiting and repairing the damage in multiple sclerosis. J Neurol Neurosurg Psychiatry 1991; 54:945-948.

86. Confavreux C, Goudable B, Moreau T.Etiologie de la sclerose en plaques. Rev Prat 1991; 41:1888-1892.

87. Consroe P, Musty R, Rein J, Tillery W, Pertwee R. The perceived effects of smoked cannabis on patients with multiple sclerosis. Eur Neurol 1997; 38: 44-48.

88. Constantinescu CS, Hilliard B, Fujioka T, Bhopale MK, Calida D, Rostami AM. Pathogenesis of neuroimmunologic diseases. Experimental models. Immunol Res 1998; 17: 217-227.

89. Cook SD, Cromarty JI, Tapp W, Poskanzer D, Walker J, Dowling PC. Declining incidence of multiple sclerosis in the Orkney Islands. Neurology 1985; 34:545-555.

90. Cook SD, Devereux C, Troiano R, Wolansky L, Guarnaccia J, Haffty B, Bansil S, Goldstein J, Sheffet A, Zito G, Jotkowitz A, Boos J, Dowling P, Rohowsky Kochan C, Volmer T. Modified total lymphoid irradiation and low dose corticosteroids in progressive multiple sclerosis. J Neurol Sci. 1997; 152: 172-181.

91. Cook SD, Dowling OC. Multiple sclerosis and viruses. Neurology 1980; 30: 80-91.

92. Cook SD, Gudmundsson G, Benedikz J, Dowling PC. Multiple sclerosis and distemper in Iceland 1966-1978. Acta Neurol Scand 1980; 61: 244-251.

93. Cook SD, MacDonald J, Tapp W, Poskanzer D, Dowling PC. Multiple sclerosis in the Shetland Islands: an update. Acta Neurol Scand 1988; 77:148-151.

94. Cook SD, Rohowsky-Kochan C, Bansil S, Dowling PC. Evidence for multiple sclerosis as an infectious disease. Acta Neurol Scand (suppl) 1995; 161: 34-42.

95. Cook SD et al. Epidemiological studies in multiple sclerosis. Neurology 1985; 35: 1528-1529.

96. Corominas J. Breve diccionario etimológico de la lengua castellana. Gredos, Madrid 1973.

97. Crawford MA, Harbige LS. The biochemical background to the integrity of the brain. En: Rose CF, Jones R (eds). Multiple sclerosis. Immunological, diagnostic and therapeutic aspects, pp 163-177. John Libbey, London 1989.

98. Cruveilhier (1835). Citado por Adams y Victor 1985.

99. Cruveilhier J. Anatomie pathologique du corps humain. JB Bailliére, Paris (1829-1842).

100. Davies JS, Hinds NP, Scanlon MF. Growth hormone deficiency and hypogonadism in a patient with multiple sclerosis. Clin Endocrinol (Oxf) 1996; 44:117-119.

101. Davis RK, Maslow AS. Multiple sclerosis in pregnancy: a review. Obstet Gynecol Surv. 1992 May. 47(5). P 290-6.

102. Dean G, Aksoy H, Akalin T, Middleton L, Kyriallis K. Multiple sclerosis in the Turkish- and Greek-speaking communities of Cyprus. A United Nations (UNHCR) Bicommunal Project. J Neurol Sci 1997; 145:163-168.

103. Dean G, Elian M. Age at immigration to England of Asian and Caribbean immigrants and the risk of developing multiple sclerosis. J Neurol Neurosurg Psychiatry 1997; 63: 565-568.

104. DeJong RN. Multiple sclerosis: history, definition and general considerations. En: Vinken PJ, Bruyn GW (ed.). Multiple sclerosis and others demyelinating diseases. Handbook of Clinical Neurology. American Elsevier Pub Co, NY 1970.

105. Demirkiran M, Jankovic J. Paroxysmal dyskinesias: clinical features and classification. Ann Neurol 1995; 38:571-579.

106. Denys P, Mane M, Azouvi P, Chartier-Kastler E, Thiebaut JB, Bussel B. Side effects of chronic intrathecal baclofen on erection and ejaculation in patients with spinal cord lesions. Arch Phys Med Rehabil 1998; 79: 494-496

107. Diana R, Grosz A, Mancini E. Personality aspects in multiple sclerosis. Ital J Neurol Sci 1985; 6:415-423.

108. Dickinson CJ. Chronic fatigue syndrome -aetiological aspects. Eur J Clin Invest 1997; 27:257-267.

109. Djaldetti R, Achiron A, Ziv I, Djaldetti M, Melamed E, Fishman P. IL-3-LA production by mononuclear cells of patients with multiple sclerosis: effect of treatment with intravenous immunoglobulins. Immunol Invest 1995; 24:765-773.

110. Donker GA, Foets M, Spreeuwenberg P, van der Steen J. [Multiple sclerosis in family practice]. Multipele sclerose in de huisartspraktijk. Ned Tijdschr Geneeskd 1996; 140:1459-1463.

111. Douglas RM, Moore BW, Miles HB. Prophylactic efficacy of intra-nasal alpha2-interferon against rhinovirus infections in the family setting. N Engl J Med 1986; 314:65-70.

112. Dousset V, Grossman RI, Ramer KN et al. Experimental allergic encephalo-myelitis and multiple sclerosis: lesion characterization with magnetization transfer imaging. Radiology 1992; 182: 483-492.

113. Dula E, Leach GE. Role of urologist in diagnosis of multiple sclerosis. Urology 1991; 37:311-313.

114. Duncan ID, Grever WE, Zhang SC. Repair of myelin disease: strategies and progress in animal models. Mol Med Today 1997; 3: 554-561

115. Duquette P, Murray TJ, Pleines J, Ebers GC, Sadovnick D, Weldon P, Warren S, Paty DW, Upton A, Hader W, et al. Multiple sclerosis in childhood: clinical profile in 125 patients. J Pediatr 1987; 111:359-363.

116. Duquette P, Pleines J, Girard M, Charest L, Senecal-Quevillon M, Masse C. The increased susceptibility of women to multiple sclerosis. Can J Neurol Sci 1992; 19:466-471.

117. Ebers GC. Immunology. En: Paty DW, Ebers GC (eds). Multiple sclerosis, pp 403-426. FA Davis Company, Philadelphia 1998

118. Ebers GC. Genetic epidemiology of multiple sclerosis. Curr Opin Neurol 1996; 9:155-158. (b)

119. Ebers GC, Bulman DE, Sadovnick AD et al. A population-based study of multiple sclerosis in twins. N Eng J Med 1986; 315: 1638-1642.

120. Edan G, Sabouraud O. Les formes benignes de sclerose en plaques. Rev Prat 1991; 41:1904-1907.

121. Edland A, Nyland H, Riise T, Larsen JP. Epidemiology of multiple sclerosis in the county of Vestfold, eastern Norway: incidence and prevalence calculations. Acta Neurol Scand 1996; 93: 104-109.

122. Elias SB. Oligodendrocyte develop-ment and the natural history of multiple sclerosis. A new hypothesis for the pathogenesis of the disease. Arch Neurol 1987; 44:1294-1299.

123. Ellison GW. Multiple sclerosis: why? Biomed Pharmacother 1989; 43:327-333.

124. Enciclopedia universal de la cultura, El Mundo. Planeta, Barcelona 1996.

125. Engell T, Trojaborg W, Raun NE. Subclinical optic neuropathy in multiple sclerosis. A neuro-ophthalmological investigation by means of visually evoked response, Farnworth-Munsell 100 Hue test and Ishihara test and their diagnostic value.Acta Ophthalmol (Copenh) 1987; 65:735-740.

126. Erkut ZA, Hofman MA, Ravid R, Swaab DF. Increased activity of hypothalamic corticotropin-releasing hor-mone neurons in multiple sclerosis. J Neuroimmunol 1995; 62:27-33.

127. Escudero D, Latorre P, Codina M, Coll-Canti J, Coll J. Central nervous system disease in Sjogren's syndrome. Ann Med Interne (Paris) 1995; 146:239-242.

128. Falcón Martínez C, Fernández-Galiano E, López Melero R. Diccionario de la mitología clásica. Alianza Editorial, Madrid 1981.

129. Fassbender K, Schmidt R, Mossner R, Kischka U, Kuhnen J, Schwartz A, Hennerici M. Mood disorders and dysfunction of the hypothalamic pituitary adrenal axis in multiple sclerosis: association with cerebral inflammation. Arch Neurol 1998; 55: 66-72

130. Fawcett J, Sidney JS, Riley-Lawless K, Hanson MJ. An exploratory study of the relationship between alternative therapies, functional status, and symptom severity among people with multiple sclerosis. J Holist Nurs 1996; 14: 115-129.

131. Fawcett J, Skegg DC. Geographic distribution of MS in New Zealand: evidence from hospital admissions and deaths. Neurology 1988; 38:416-418.

132. Fazekas F, Deisenhammer F, Strasser-Fuschs S, Nahler G, Mamoli B. Randomized placebo-controlled trial of monthly intravenous immunoglobulin therapy in relapsing-remitting multiple sclerosis. Austroian Immunoglobulin in multiple sclerosis study group. Lancet 1997; 349:589-593.

133. Fazekas F, Deisenhammer F, Strasser-Fuschs S, Nahler G, Mamoli B. Treatment effects of monthly intravenous immunoglobulin on patients with relapsing-remitting multiple sclerosis: further analyses of the Austrian Immunoglobulin in MS study. Mult Scler 1997; 3:137-141.

134. Feinstein A, Feinstein K, Gray T, O' Connor P. Prevalence and neurobehavioral correlates of pathological laughing and crying in multiple sclerosis. Arch Neurol 1997; 54: 1116-1121.

135. Felgenhauer K. Psychiatric disorders in the encephalitic form of multiple sclerosis. J Neurol 1990; 237:11-18.

136. Ferini-Strambi L, Filippi M, Martinelli V, Oldani A, Rovaris M, Zucconi M, Comi G, Smirne S. Nocturnal sleep study in multiple sclerosis: correlations with clinical and brain magnetic resonance imaging findings. J Neurol Sci 1994; 125:194-197.

137. Ferini-Strambi L, Smirne S. Cardiac autonomic function during sleep in several neuropsychiatric disorders. J Neurol 1997; 244(Suppl 1):S29-36.

138. Fernández Fernández Ó. Epidemio-logía de la esclerosis múltiple en España. En: Alfaro A, Palao A, Sancho J (eds): Neuroepidemiología (pp 115-122), MCR SA, Barcelona 1990.

139. Fernández Fernández Ó. Esclerosis múltiple: una aproximación multidisci-plinaria. Arké 144 SL, Madrid 1994.

140. Fernández Fernández Ó. Tratamiento de la esclerosis múltiple: puesta al día. Boletín Terapéutico Andaluz 1997; 13:17-20.

141. Fernández Fernández O, Fernández VE . Esclerosis múltiple: una enfermedad relativamente frecuente en España. Alphagraphics, Málaga 1996.

142. Fernández Fernández Ó, Fernández VE . Esclerosis múltiple: una enfermedad relativamente frecuente en España. Alphagraphics, Málaga 1997 (2ª edición).

143. Fernandez Fernández O, Izquierdo G, Campos VM, Pastor M. Epidemiología de la esclerosis multiple en la provincia de Malaga (España). Un estudio de prevalencia. Neurología 1986; 1:3-5.

144. Fernández Fernández Ó, Luque G, San Román C, Bravo M, Dean G. The prevalence of multiple sclerosis in the sanitary district of Vélez Málaga, southern Spain. Neurology 1994; 44:425-429.

145. Fernández Uriel P, Vázquez Hoys AM. Diccionario del mundo antiguo. Alianza Editorial, Madrid 1994.

146. Filipovic SR, Drulovic J, Stojsavljevic N, Levic Z. The effects of high dose intravenous methylprednisolone on event related potentials in patients with multiple sclerosis. J Neurol Sci 1997; 152: 147-153

147. Filippi M, Paty DW, Kappos L et al. Correlations between changes in disability and T2-weighted brain MRI activity in multiple sclerosis: a follow-up study. Neurology 1995; 45: 255-260.

148. Filley CM, Heaton RK, Nelson LM, Burks JS, Franklin GM. A comparison of dementia in Alzheimer's disease and multiple sclerosis. Arch Neurol 1989; 46:157-161.

149. Finger S. A happy state of mind: a history of mild elation, denial of disability, optimism, and laughing in multiple sclerosis. Arch Neurol 1998; 55: 241-250

150. Firth D. The case of Augustus D'Esté. Cambridge University Press, London 1948.

151. Fischer JS, Cleveland OH, Priore R, Jacobs L et al. Neuropsychological effects of Avonex (interferon-beta1a) in relapsing multiple sclerosis. 50th Annual Meeting American Academy of Neurology, Minneapolis April 25-May 2, 1998.

152. Fisher M, Johnson MH, Natale AM, Levine PH. Linoleic acid levels in white blood cells, platelets, and serum of multiple sclerosis patients. Acta Neurol Scand 1987; 76:241-245.

153. Flint S, Scully C. Isolated trigeminal sensory neuropathy: a heterogeneous group of disorders. Oral Surg Oral Med Oral Pathol 1990; 69:153-156.

154. Fog T. ACTH therapy of multiple sclerosis. Nord Med 1951; 46: 1742-1748.

155. Foley FW, Werner MA. Sexuality. En: Kalb RC (ed). Multiple sclerosis. The questions you have, the answers you need, pp 223-247. Demos Vermande, New York 1996.

156. Foong J, Rozewicz L, Quaghebeur G, Thompson AJ, Miller DH, Ron MA. Neuropsychological deficits in multiple sclerosis after acute relapse. J Neurol Neurosurg Psychiatry 1998; 64: 529-532

157. Ford B, Tampieri D, Francis G. Long-term follow-up of acute partial transverse myelopathy. Neurology 1992; 42:250-252.

158. Foster V, MacFarlane EB. Clear thinking about alternatives therapies. National Multiple Sclerosis Society, New York 1996.

159. Fowler CV. Bladder dysfunction in multiple sclerosis: causes and treatment. Int MSJ 1994; 1:99-107.

160. Foucault M. Les mots et les choses. Une archéologie des sciences humaines. Gallimard, Paris 1966.

161. Frank C. Psychische Veranderungen bei Multipler Sklerose. Wien Med Wochenschr 1985; 135:12-17.

162. Frankel D, Jones H. Living with MS. National Multiple Sclerosis Society, New York 1998.

163. Frederiksen JL. Optic neuritis: a common first manifestation of multiple sclerosis. Int MSJ 1995; 2: 27-32.

164. Freedman MS, Gray TA. Vascular headache: a presenting symptom of multiple sclerosis. Can J Neurol Sci 1989; 16:63-66.
165. Frerichs FT. Über Hirnsklerose. Arch Ges Med 1849; 10:334-337

166. Freud. Estudios sobre la histeria (1895). Obras completas. Biblioteca Nueva, Madrid 1973.

167. Fricker J. Developing drugs for multiple sclerosis (editorial). Lancet 1996; 348:1022.

168. Gale CR, Martyn CN. Migrant studies in multiple sclerosis. Prog Neurobiol 1995; 47:425-448.

169. García-Monco JC, Miro Jornet J, Fernández Villar B; Benach JL, Guerrero Espejo A, Berciano JA. Esclerosis múltiple o enfermedad de Lyme? Un problema diagnóstico de exclusion. Med Clin (Barc) 1990; 94:685-688.

170. Gasperini C, Grasso MG, Fiorelli M, Millefiorini E, Morino S, Anzini A, Colleluori A, Salvetti M, Buttinelli C, Pozzilli C. A controlled study of potential risk factors preceding exacerbation in multiple sclerosis. J Neurol Neurosurg Psychiatry 1995; 59:303-305.

171. Gidal BE et al. Current developments in Neurology, part I. Advances in the pharmacotherapy of headache, epilepsy, and multiple sclerosis. Ann Pharmacother 1996; 30:1272-1276.

172. Gilbert JJ, Sadler M. Unsuspected multiple sclerosis. Arch Neurol 1983; 40: 533.

173. Giubilei F, Vitale A, Urani C, Frontoni M, Fiorini M, Millefiorini E, Fiorelli M, Santini M, Strano S. Cardiac autonomic dysfunction in relapsing-remitting multiple sclerosis during a stable phase. Eur Neurol 1996; 36:211-214.

174. Glaser GH, Merritt HH. Effects of corticotrophin (ACTH) and cortisone on disorders of the nervous system. JAMA 1952; 148: 898.

175. Goldberg P, Fleming MC, Picard EH. Multiple sclerosis: decreased relapse rate through dietary supplementation with calcium, magnesium and vitamin D. Med Hypotheses 1986; 21:193-200.

176. González CF, Swirsky-Sacchetti T, Mitchell D, Lublin FD, Knobler RL, Ehrlich SM. Distributional patterns of multiple sclerosis brain lesions. Magnetic resonance imaging--clinical correlation. J Neuroimaging 1994; 4: 188-195.

177. González Maldonado R. El extraño caso del Dr. Parkinson (4ª ed.) Grupo Editorial Universitario, Granada 1997.

178. González Maldonado R et al. Corea paroxística en esclerosis múltiple. Comunicación a la Reunión Ordinaria de la Sociedad Andaluza de Neurología, Granada 1991.*

179. González Maldonado R, Moreno Alegre V, Juma Mentado C, Moldenhauer JF. Consideraciones etiopatogénicas, clínicas y terapéuticas del síndrome de Gélineau. Phronesis 1980; 6:353-361.

180. Good DM, Bower DA, Einsporn RL. Social support: gender differences in multiple sclerosis spousal caregivers. J Neurosci Nurs 1995; 27: 305-311.

181. Goodkin DE, Rudick RA. Multiple sclerosis. Advances in clinical trial design, treatment and future perspectives. Springer, London 1996.

182. Goodwin SD, Sproat TT, Russell WL. Management of Lyme disease.
183. Clin Pharm 1990; 9: 192-205.

184. Gottlieb SF, Smith JE, Neubauer RA. The etiology of multiple sclerosis: a new and extended vascular-ischemic model. Med Hypotheses 1990; 33:23-29.

185. Gracia F, Castillo L, de Lao SL, Archibold CA, Larreategui M, Reeves WC, Levine P. Enfermedades neurologicas asociadas al virus HTLV-1 en Panama. Rev Med Panama 1990; 15:197-203.

186. Gracián B. Oráculo manual y arte de prudencia (1647). Obras completas. Aguilar, Madrid 1967.

187. Granieri E, Malagu S, Casetta I, Tola MR, Govoni V, Paolino E, Monetti VC. Multiple sclerosis in Italy. A reappraisal of incidence and prevalence in Ferrara. Arch Neurol 1996; 53:793-798.

188. Grant I. The social environment and neurological disease. Adv Psychosom Med 1985; 13:26-48.

189. Grant I. Neuropsychological and psychiatric distubances in multiple sclerosis. En: McDonald WI, Silberberg DH (eds). Multiple sclerosis, pp 134-152. Butterworths, London 1986.

190. Grant I, McDonald WI, Patterson TL, Trimble MR. Multiple sclerosis. En: Brown GW, Harris T (eds): Life events and illness: studies of psychiatryc and physical disorders, pp 295-311. Guilford Press, New York 1989.

191. Graves R. Los mitos griegos (vol. 1 y 2). Alianza Editorial, Madrid 1986.

192. Greenberg SJ. Human retroviruses and demyelinating diseases. Neurol Clin 1995; 13:75-97. (a)
193. Greenberg SJ. Retrovirus humanos y enfermedades desmielinizantes. En: Antel JP. Esclerosis múltiple. Clínicas Neurológicas de Norteamérica, 1995; 1:1-21. (b)

194. Greer R. Diets to help multiple sclerosis. Harper Collins Publishers, London 1995.

195. Gruener DM, Kunkel EJ, Snyderman DA, Infante MR, Rodgers C, Field HL. Dietary vitamin B12 deficiency in a patient with multiple sclerosis. Gen Hosp Psychiatry 1994; 16:224-228.

196. Gusev E, Boiko A, Lauer K, Riise T, Deomina T. Environmental risk factors in MS: a case-control study in Moscow. Acta Neurol Scand 1996; 94: 386-394.

197. Guthrie TC, Nelson DA.Influence of temperature changes on multiple sclerosis: critical review of mechanisms and research potential. J Neurol Sci 1995; 129:1-8.
198. Hader WJ, Irvine DG, Schiefer HB. A cluster-focus of multiple sclerosis at Henribourg, Saskatchewan. Can J Neurol Sci 1990; 17:391-4.

199. Hainsworth MA. Living with multiple sclerosis: the experience of chronic sorrow. J Neurosci Nurs 1994; 26:237-240.

200. Hainsworth MA, Burke ML, Lindgren CL, Eakes GG. Home Healthc Nurse 1993; 11:9-13.

201. Hammond A. A treatise on diseases of the nervous system. D. Appleton & Co, New York 1871.

202. Hammond SR, de Wytt C, Maxwell IC, Landy PJ, English D, McLeod JG, McCall MG. The epidemiology of multiple sclerosis in Queensland, Australia. J Neurol Sci 1987; 80:185-204.

203. Harbison JW, Calabrese VP, Edlich RF. A fatal case of sun exposure in a multiple sclerosis patient. J Emerg Med 1989; 7:465-467.
204. Harris JO, Frank JA, Patronas N et al. Serial gadolinium-enhanced magnetic resonance imaging scans in patients with early, relapsing-remitting multiple sclerosis: implications for clinical trials and natural history. Ann Neurol 1991; 29: 548-555.

205. Hauser SL. Why study genes? Inside MS 1998; 1:44-47.

206. Hayden FG, Albrecht JK, Kaiser DL, Gwaltney JM Jr. Prevention of natural cold by contact prophylaxys with intranasal alpha-interferon. N Engl J Med 1986; 314:71-75.

207. Heaton RK, Nelson LM, Thompson DS et al. Neuropsychological findings in relapsing-remitting and chronic-progressive multiple sclerosis. J Consult Clin Psychol 1985; 53:103.

208. Heinsen H, Lockemann U, Puschel K. Unsuspected (clinically silent) multiple sclerosis. Quantitative investigations in one autoptic case. Int J Legal Med 1995; 107: 263-266.

209. Helmick CG, Wrigley JM, Zack MM, Bigler WJ, Lehman JL, Janssen RS, Hartwig EC, Witte JJ. Multiple sclerosis in Key West, Florida. Am J Epidemiol. 1989 Nov. 130(5). P 935-49.

210. Heltberg A. Twin studies in multiple sclerosis. Ital J Neurol Sci 1987; Suppl 6:35-39.

211. Henze T, Prange HW, Talartschik J, Rumpf KW. Complications of plasma exchange in patients with neurological diseases. Klin Wochenschr 1990; 68:1183-1188.

212. Hernández Pérez MA, Fernández Fernández O. Nuevas perspectivas en el diagnóstico de la esclerosis múltiple. JR Prous, Barcelona 1994.

213. Herrera WG. Vestibular and other balance disorders in multiple sclerosis. Differential diagnosis of disequilibrium and topognostic localization. Neurol Clin 1990; 8:407-420.

214. Hertz L, McFarlin DE, Waksman BH. Astrocytes: auxiliary cells for immune responses in the central nervous system? Immunol Today 1990; 11:265-268.

215. Hewer W, Junker D, Dressing H, Olbrich R. Psychosen bei Enzephalitiden unklarer Atiologie. Atypische Verlaufsfor-men einer Multiplen Sklerose? Nervenarzt 1994; 65:163-168.

216. Hibbeln JR, Salem N Jr. Dietary polyunsaturated fatty acids and depression: when cholesterol does not satisfy. Am J Clin Nutr 1995; 62:1-9.

217. Hohol MJ, Khoury SJ, Cook SL, Orav EJ, Hafler DA, Weiner HL. Three-year open protocol continuation study of oral tolerization with myelin antigens in multiple sclerosis and design of a phase III pivotal trial. Ann N Y Acad Sci 1996; 13:243-250.

218. Holland NJ, Stockwell S. Controlling spasticity. National Multiple Sclerosis Society, New York 1998.

219. Hommes OR, Barkhof F, Jongen PJ, Frequin ST. Methylprednisolone treatment in multiple sclerosis: effect of treatment, pharmacokinetics, future. Mult Scler 1996; 1: 327-328.

220. Honer WG, Hurwitz T, Li DK, Palmer M, Paty DW. Temporal lobe involvement in multiple sclerosis patients with psychiatric disorders. Arch Neurol 1987; 44:187-190.

221. Hopkins RS, Indian RW, Pinnow E, Conomy J. Multiple sclerosis in Galion, Ohio: prevalence and results of a case-control study. Neuroepidemiology 1991; 10:192-199.

222. Houtchens MK, Richert JR, Sami A, Rose JW. Open label gabapentin treatment for pain in multiple sclerosis. Mult Scler 1997; 3: 250-253.

223. Hoyo A. Diccionario de palabras y frases extranjeras. Aguilar, Madrid 1988.

224. Hutchinson M. Pregnancy in multiple sclerosis. Int MSJ 1996; 3:81-84.

225. Hutchinson M, Stack J, Buckley P. Bipolar affective disorder prior to the onset of multiple sclerosis. Acta Neurol Scand 1993; 88:388-393.

226. Hutter CD, Laing P. Multiple sclerosis: sunlight, diet, immunology and aetiology. Med Hypotheses 1996; 46: 67-74.

227. Huws R, Shubsachs AP, Taylor PJ. Hypersexuality, fetishism and multiple sclerosis. Br J Psychiatry 1991; 158:280-281.

228. IFNB Multiple Sclerosis Study Group. Interferon beta-1b is effective in relapsing-remitting multiple sclerosis. I. Clinical results of a multicenter, randomized, double-blind, placebo-controlled trial. Neurology 1993; 43: 655-661.

229. IFNB Multiple Sclerosis Study Group. Treatment of MS with interferon beta-1b -fnal clinical results of the betaseron trial. Ivth International Congress of Neuroimmunology, the Netherlands, October 1994. J Immunol 1994; 54:178.

230. IFNB Multiple Sclerosis Study Group and the University of British Columbia MS/MRI Analysis Group: Interferon beta-1b in the treatment of multiple sclerosis: Final outcome of the randomized controlled trial. Neurology 1995; 45: 1277-1285.

231. IFNB Multiple Sclerosis Study Group and the University of British Columbia MS/MRI Analysis Group: Neutralizing antibodies during treatment of of multiple sclerosis with interferon beta-1b: Experience during the first three years. Neurology 1996; 47: 889-894.

232. Ivnik RJ. Neuropsychological stability in multiple sclerosis. J Consult Clin Psychol 1978; 46: 913-923.

233. Izquierdo G, Lyon-Caen O, Marteau R, Martinez-Parra C, Lhermitte F, Castaigne P, Hauw JJ. Early onset multiple sclerosis. Clinical study of 12 patholo-gically proven cases. Acta Neurol Scand 1986; 73:493-497.

234. Jacobs LD et al. The Multiple Sclerosis Collaborative Research Group. Intramuscular interferon beta-1a for disease pregression in relapsing multiple sclerosis. Ann Neurology 1996; 39:285-294.

235. Jacobson S, Zaninovic V, Mora C, Rodgers-Johnson P, Sheremata WA, Gibbs CJ Jr; Gajdusek C; McFarlin DE. Immunological findings in neurological diseases associated with antibodies to HTLV-I: activated lymphocytes in tropical spastic paraparesis. Ann Neurol 1988: 23 (suppl):S196-200.

236. Jacome DE. La toux diabolique: neurogenic tussive crisis. Postgrad Med J 1985; 61:515-516.

237. Jaworski MA, Severini A, Mansour G, Hennig K, Slater JD, Jeske R, Schlaut J, Yoon JW, Maclaren NK, Nepom GT. Inherited diseases in North American Mennonites: focus on Old Colony (Chortitza) Mennonites. Am J Med Genet 1989; 32: 158-168.

238. Jellinek EH. Heine's illness: the case for multiple sclerosis. JR Soc Med 1990; 83: 516-519.

239. Jennekins-Schinkel A, Laboyrie PM, Lanser JBK, van der Velde EA. Cognition in patients with multiple sclerosis: after four years. J Neurol Sci 1990; 99: 229-247.

240. Joffe RT, Lippert GP, Gray TA, Sawa G, Horvath Z. Mood disorder and multiple sclerosis. Arch Neurol 1987; 44:376-378. (a)

241. Joffe RT, Lippert GP, Gray TA, Sawa G, Horvath Z. Personal and family history of affective illness in patients with multiple sclerosis. J Affect Disord 1987; 12:63-65.(b)

242. Johnson RT. The virology of demyelinating diseases. Ann Neurol 1994; 36(Suppl):S54-60.

243. Juan. Evangelio, 13-27. Nuevo Testa-mento. Santa Biblia. Planeta, Barcelona 1961.

244. Jung CG. Formaciones de lo inconsciente. Paidós Ibérica, Barcelona 1992.

245. Kadish U, Gadoth N. [Heinrich Heine - death of a poet]. Harefuah 1995; 128: 391-393.

246. Kahana E, Leibowitz V, Alter M. Cerebral multiple sclerosis. Neurology 1971; 21:1179.

247. Kahana E, Zilber N, Abramson JH, Biton V, Leibowitz Y, Abramsky O. Multiple sclerosis: genetic versus environmental aetiology: epidemiology in Israel updated. J Neurol 1994; 241:341-346.

248. Kalafatova OI. Epidemiology of multiple sclerosis in Bulgaria. Acta Neurol Scand 1987; 75:186-189.

249. Kalb RC (ed). Multiple sclerosis. The questions you have, the answers you need. Demos Vermande, New York 1996. (*passim*)

250. Karussis DM, Meiner Z, Lechmann D, Gomori JM, Scharz A, Linde A, Abramsky O. Treatment of secondary progresive multiple sclerosis with the immuno-modulator linomide: a double-blind, placebo-controlled pilot study sith monthly magnetic resonance imaging evaluation. Neurology 1996; 47: 341-346.

251. Kavafis K. Poesías completas. Orbis, Barcelona 1997.

252. Kesselring J. Die Prognose der Multi-plen Sklerose. Schweiz Med Wochenschr 1997; 127: 500-505.

253. Kesselring J. Multiple sclerosis. Cambridge University Press, Cambridge 1997. (*passim*)

254. Khodos KhG, Kozhova II, Berdennikova VV. [The role of functional disorders of the autonomic nervous system in the pathogenesis of multiple sclerosis]. O znachenii disfunktsii vegetativnoi nervnoi sistemy v patogeneze rasseiannogo skleroza. Zh Nevropatol Psikhiatr Im S S Korsakova 1990; 90:112-115.

255. Kibler RF. Large dose corticosteroid therapy of experimental and human demyelinating diseases. NY Acad Sci 1965; 122: 469-479.

256. Kibler RF, Paty DW, Re PK, McPhedran AM, Karp HR. Effect of large doses of adrenocrticosteroids on the course of EAE and multiple sclerosis. En: Wolfgram F, Ellison GW, Stevens JG, Andrews DM (eds): Multiple sclerosis. Immunology, virology and ultra structure, pp 511-529. Academic Press, New York 1972.

257. Kinnunen E, Juntunen J, Ketonen L, Koskimies S, Konttinen YT, Salmi T, Koskenvuo M, Kaprio J. Genetic susceptibility to multiple sclerosis. A co-twin study of a nationwide series. Arch Neurol 1988; 45:1108-1111.

258. Kirkeby HJ, Poulsen EU, Petersen T, Dorup J. Erectile dysfunction in multiple sclerosis. Neurology 1988; 38:1366-1371.

259. Klonoff HH, Clark C, Oger JJF, Paty DW, Li DKB. Neuropsychological performance in patients with mild multiple sclerosis. J Nerv Ment Dis 1991; 179: 127-131.

260. Knorr-Held S, Brendel W, Kiefer H, Paal G, von Specht BU. Sensitization against brain gangliosides after therapeutic swine brain implantation in a multiple sclerosis patient. J Neurol 1986; 233:54-56.

261. Koopmans RA, Li DK, Grochowski E, Cutler PJ, Paty DW. Benign versus chronic progressive multiple sclerosis: magnetic resonance imaging features. Ann Neurol 1989; 25:74-81.

262. Koprowski H, DeFreitas E. HTLV-I and chronic nervous diseases: present status and a look into the future. Ann Neurol 1988; 23 (suppl):166-170.

263. Korn-Lubetzki I, Kahana E, Cooper G, Abramsky O. Activity of multiple sclerosis during pregnancy and puerperium. Ann Neurol 1984; 16: 229-231.

264. Kraft G, Alquist A. Effect os microclimate cooling on physical function in multiple sclerosis. Multiple Sclerosis Association of America, Cherry Hill, NJ 1997.

265. Krupp LB, Coyle PK, Doscher C, Miller A, Cross AH, Jandorf L, Halper J, Johnson B, Morgante L, Grimson R. Fatigue therapy in multiple sclerosis: results of a double-blind,randomized, parallel trial of amantadine, pemoline, and placebo. Neurology 1995; 45:1956-1961.

266. Kuhn TS. La estructura de las revoluciones científicas. Fondo de cultura económica, Madrid 1997.

267. Kuppersmith MJ, Kaufman D, Paty DW et al. Megadose corticosteroids in multiple sclerosis. Neurology 1994; 44: 1-4.

268. Kurtzke JF. Multiple sclerosis: changing times (editorial). Neuroepi-demiology 1991; 10:1-8.

269. Kurtzke JF, Beebe GW, Nagler B et al. Studies on the natural history of multiple sclerosis 6. Clinical and laboratory findings at first diagnosis. Acta Neurol Scand 1972; 48-19.

270. Kurtzke JF; Beebe GW; Norman JE Jr. Epidemiology of multiple sclerosis in US veterans: III. Migration and the risk of MS. Neurology. 1985; 35:672-8.

271. Kurtzke JF, Gudmundsson KR, Bergmann S. Multiple sclerosis in Iceland. 1: Evidence of a post-war epidemic. Neurology 1982; 32:143.

272. Kurtzke JF, Hyllested K. Multiple sclerosis in the Faroe Islands. 1: Clinical and epidemiological features. Ann Neurol 1979; 5: 6.

273. Kurtzke JF, Hyllested K. Multiple sclerosis epidemiology in Faroe Islands. Riv Neurol 1987; 57: 77-87.

274. Kurtzke JF, Page WF. Epidemiology of multiple sclerosis in US veterans: VII. Risk factors for MS. Neurology 1997; 48: 204-213.

275. Kurtzke JF, Page WF, Murphy FM, Norman JE Jr. Epidemiology of multiple sclerosis in US veterans. 4. Age at onset. Neuroepidemiology 1992; 11: 226-235.

276. Labarrere CA, Catoggio LJ, Mullen EG, Althabe OH. Placental lesions in maternal autoimmune diseases. Am J Reprod Immunol Microbiol 1986; 12:78-86.

277. Laborde JM, Dando WA, Teetzen ML. Climate, diffused solar radiation and multiple sclerosis. Soc Sci Med 1988; 27:231-238.

278. LaRocca NG, Fisher J. Stress and emotional issues. En: Kalb RC (ed). Multiple sclerosis. The questions you have, the answers you need, pp 205-221. Demos Vermande, New York 1996.

279. LaRocca NG, King M. Solving cognitive problems. National Multiple Sclerosis Society, New York 1998.

280. Larsen JP, Kvaale G, Riise T, Nyland H, Aarli JA. Multiple sclerosis -more than one disease? Acta Neurol Scand 1985; 72:145-150.

281. Larsson HB, Stubgaard M, Frederiksen JL, Jensen M, Henriksen O, Paulson OB. Quantitation of blood-brain barrier defect by magnetic resonance imaging and gadolinium-DTPA in patients with multiple sclerosis and brain tumors. Magn Reson Med 1990; 16:117-31.

282. Lauer K. Dietary changes in temporal relation to multiple sclerosis in the Faroe Islands: an evaluation of literary sources. Neuroepidemiology. 1989. 8(4). P 200-6. (a)

283. Lauer K. Multiple sclerosis in relation to meat preservation in France and Switzerland. Neuroepidemiology 1989; 8:308-315. (b)

284. Lauer K. Mortality of multiple sclerosis in relation to geographic factors in France. Neuroepidemiology 1990; 9:113-117.

285. Lauer K. The history of nitrite in human nutrition: a contribution from German cookery books. J Clin Epidemiol 1991; 44:261-264.

286. Lauer K. The risk of multiple sclerosis in the U.S.A. in relation to sociogeographic features: a factor-analytic study. J Clin Epidemiol 1994; 47:43-48.

287. Lauer K, Firnhaber W. Epidemiological investigations into multiple sclerosis in Southern Hesse. III. The possible influence of occupation on the risk of disease. Acta Neurol Scand 1985; 72:397-402.

288. Lauer K, Firnhaber W. Epidemio-logische Aspekte der multiplen Sklerose. Versicherungsmedizin. 1992 Aug 1. 44(4). P 125-30.

289. Lázaro Carreter F. El dardo en la palabra. Galaxia Gutenberg, Círculo de lectores, Barcelona 1997.

290. Lechtenberg R. Multiple Sclerosis, Fact Book. FA Davis, Philadelphia 1995.

291. Lee KH, Hashimoto SA, Hodge JP et al. MRI of the head in the diagnosis of multiple sclerosis: A prospective 2-year follow-up with comparison with clinical evaluation, evoked potentials, oligoclonal banding, and CT. Neurology 1991; 41:657-660.

292. Lehmann D, Ben-Nun A. Bacterial agents protect against autoimmune disease. I. Mice pre-exposed to Bordetella pertussis or Mycobacterium tuberculosis are highly refractory to induction of experimental autoimmune encephalomyelitis. J Autoimmun 1992; 5:675-690.

293. Leibowitz U, Kahana E, Alter M. Multiple sclerosis in immigrant and native populations of Israel. Lancet 1970; 1:1323-1325.

294. Lengdobler H, Kiessling WR. [Group music therapy in multiple sclerosis: initial report of experience]. Psychoter Psychosom Med Psychol 1989; 39: 369-373.

295. Lensky P. [Geographic aspects in the epidemiology of multiple sclerosis]. Geograficky aspekt v epidemiologii sclerosis multiplex. Epidemiol Mikrobiol Imunol 1994; 43: 174-176.

296. Lévy H. Entrevistado por Lluís Reales en "La Vanguardia". Barcelona, 7 marzo 1998.

297. Libenson MH, Stafstrom CE, Rosman NP. Tonic "seizures" in a patient with brainstem demyelination: MRI study of brain and spinal cord. Pediatr Neurol 1994; 11:258-262.

298. Liu X, Linnington C, Webster HF, Lassmann S, Yao DL, Hudson LD, Wekerle H, Kreutzberg GW. Insulin-like growth factor-I treatment reduces immune cell responses in acute non-demyelinative experimental autoimmune encephalo-myelitis. J Neuroscienc Res 1997; 47: 531-538.

299. Liu M, Xu W. [Practical value of IgG index and IgG synthesis rate in multiple sclerosis]. Hua Hsi I Ko Ta Hsueh Hsueh Pao 1994; 25: 215-217.

300. Liveson JA. Peripheral Neurology. Case studies in electrodiagnosis. FA Davis Co, Philadelphia 1991.

301. Longo WE, Ballantyne GH, Modlin IM. Colorectal disease in spinal cord patients. An occult diagnosis. Dis Colon Rectum 1990; 33:131-134.

302. Lorcerie B, Marchal G, Borsotti JP, Guard O, Giroud M, Dumas R, Martin F. Sclerose en plaques associee a une symptomatologie biologique evocatrice d'un lupus erythemateux dissemine. Une observation avec étude anatomique. Rev Med Interne 1989; 10:471-474.

303. Lowis GW. The social epidemiology of disease with particular emphasis on multiple sclerosis. Sci Total Environ 1992; 126:139-164.

304. Lublin FD. Relapsing experimental allergic encephalomyelitis. An autoimmune model of multiple sclerosis. Springer Semin Immunopathol 1985; 8:197-208.

305. Lublin FD, Whitaker JN, Eidelman BH, Miller AE, Arnason BGW, Burks JS. Management of patients receiving interferon beta-1b for multiple sclerosis. Report of a consensus conference. Neurology 1996; 45: 12-18.

306. Lynch SG, Rose JW, Smoker W, Petajan JH. MRI in familial multiple sclerosis. Neurology 1990; 40:900-903.

307. MacGregor HS, Latiwonk QI. Complex role of gamma-herpesviruses in multiple sclerosis and infectious mononucleosis. Neurol Res 1993; 15: 391-394.

308. Macchi G. Experimental patterns related to multiple sclerosis pathology. Riv Neurol 1987; 57:145-153.

309. Machado A. Antología poética. Austral, Madrid 1975.*

310. Mahler ME. Behavioral manifestations associated with multiple sclerosis. Psychiatr Clin North Am 1992; 15: 427-438.

311. Malmgren RM, Dudley JP, Visscher BR, Valdiviezo NL, Clark VA, Deterls R. Mortality in persons with multiple sclerosis in the Seattle and Los Angeles areas. JAMA 1981; 246: 2042-2046.

312. Malmgren RM, Valdiviezo NL, Visscher BR et al. Underlying cause of death as recorded for multiple sclerosis patients: associated factors. J Chron Dis 1983; 36: 699-705.

313. Malosse D, Perron H, Sasco A, Seigneurin JM. Correlation between milk and dairy product consumption and multiple sclerosis prevalence: a worldwide study. Neuroepidemiology 1992; 11: 304-312.

314. Mandel AR, Keller SM. Stress management in rehabilitation. Arch Phys Med Rehabil 1986; 67:375-379.

315. Marburg O. Die sogenannte akute Multiple Sklerose. Jahrb Psychiatrie 1906; 27:211-312.

316. Martí-Fábregas J, Martínez JM, Illa I, Escartin A. Myelopathy of unknown etiology. A clinical follow-up and MRI study of 57 cases. Acta Neurol Scand 1989; 80:455-460.

317. Martin R, McFarland HF. Immuno-logical aspects of experimental allergic encephalomyelitis and multiple sclerosis. Crit Rev Clin Lab Sci 1995; 32:121-82.

318. Martin R, Matias-Guiu J, Molto JM, Insa R, Falip R, Oltra A. Epidemiología de la esclerosis multiple en el area sanitaria de Alcoy: influencia del grupo sanguíneo. Neurología 1989; 4:301-302.

319. Martinovic Z, Ristanovic D, Jovanovic V. Some uses of visual evoked potentials in the diagnostics of neurological disorders in developmental period. Neurologija 1989; 38:295-310.

320. Martyn CN. Childhood infection and adult disease. Ciba Found Symp. 1991; 156: 93-102.

321. Mascarella JJ, Hudson DC. Dysimmune neurologic disorders. AACN Clin Issues Crit Care Nurs 1991; 2:675-684.

322. Masjuan J, Buisan J, Gimeno A, Álva-rez Cermeno JC. Discinesias paroxísticas como manifestación inicial de la esclerosis multiple. Neurología. 1998; 13: 45-48

323. Matías-Guiu J. Neuroepidemiología. JR Prous, Barcelona 1993.

324. Matthews WB. Clinical aspects. En Matthews WB, Compston A, Allen IV, Martyn CN (eds). Mc Alpine's Multiple Sclerosis, pp 231-250. Churchill Livingstone, London 1991.

325. Mattson D, Petrie M, Srivastava DK, McDermott M. Multiple sclerosis. Sexual dysfunction and its response to medication. Arch Neurol 1995; 52: 862-868.

326. McAlpine D, Lumsden CE, Acheson ED. Multiple sclerosis: a reappraisal. Churchill-Livingstone, Edimburgh 1972.

327. McDonald WI. The dynamics of multiple sclerosis. The Charcot Lecture. J Neurol 1993; 240:28-36.

328. McDonald WI, Miller DH, Thompson AJ. Are magnetic resonance findings predictive of clinical outcome in therapeutic trials in multiple sclerosis? The dilemma of interferon-beta. Ann Neurol 1994; 36: 14-18.

329. McDonald WI, Miller DH, Barnes D. The pathological evolution of multiple sclerosis. Neuropathol Appl Neurobiol 1992; 18: 319-334.

330. McDonnell GV, Hawkins SA. An epidemiologic study of multiple sclerosis in Northern Ireland. Neurology 1998; 50: 423-428

331. McFarland HF, Frank JA, Albert PS et al. Using Gadolinium-enhanced magnetic resonance imaging lesions to monitor disease activity in multiple sclerosis. Ann Neurol 1992; 23: 758-766.

332. McKahn GM. Multiple sclerosis. Ann Rev Neurosci 1982; 5:219.

333. McHatters GR, Scham RG. Bird viruses in multiple sclerosis: combination of viruses or Marek's alone? Neurosci Lett 1995; 188: 75-76.

334. McLeod JG, Hammond SR, Hallpike JF. Epidemiology of multiple sclerosis in Australia. With NSW and SA survey results. Med J Aust 1994; 160:117-122.

335. McMichael AJ, Hall AJ. Does immunosuppressive ultraviolet radiation explain the latitude gradient for multiple sclerosis? Epidemiology 1997; 8: 642-645.

336. Medaer R. Does the history of multiple sclerosis go back as far as the 14th century? Acta Neurol Scand 1979; 60: 189-192.

337. Midgard R, Riise T, Svanes C, Kvale G, Nyland H. Incidence of multiple sclerosis in More and Romsdal, Norway from 1950 to 1991. An age-period-cohort analysis. Brain 1996; 119:203-211.

338. Millar JHD, Allison RS, Cheesman EA, Merrett JD. Pregnancy as a factor influencing relapse in disseminated sclerosis. Brain 1959; 82: 417-426.

339. Miller A. Current and investigational therapies used to alter the course of disease in multiple sclerosis. South Med J 1997; 90:367-375. (a)

340. Miller DH. Magnetic resonance in monitoring the treatment of multiple sclerosis. Ann Neurol 1994; 36 (suppl): S91-94.

341. Miller DH. Demyelinating diseases. Editorial comment. Current Opinion in Neurology 1997; 10:179-180. (b)

342. Miller DJ, Asakura K, Rodríguez M. Experimental strategies to promote central nervous system remyelination in multiple sclerosis: insights gained from the Theiler's virus model. J Neurosc Res 1995; 41: 291-296.

343. Miller H, Ridley A, Schapira K. Multiple sclerosis: a note on social class. Br Med J 1960; 2: 343-345.

344. Minderhoud JM, van der Hoeven JH, Prange AJ. Course and prognosis of chronic progressive multiple sclerosis. Results of an epidemiological study. Acta Neurol Scand 1988; 78:10-15.

345. Mititelu G, Bourceanu I. [Possible involvement of the canine distemper virus in the epidemiology of multiple sclerosis]. Posibila implicatie a virusului distemper canin in epidemiologia sclerozei multiple. Rev Med Chir Soc Med Nat Iasi 1985; 89:451-453. (a)

346. Mititelu G; Bourceanu I. Retrospec-tive epidemiology in multiple sclerosis and significance of canine morbillivirus in the illness etiology. Neurol Psychiatr (Bucur) 1985; 23:59-63. (b)

347. Modrego Pardo PJ, Latorre MA, Lopez A, Errea JM. Prevalence of multiple sclerosis in the province of Teruel, Spain. J Neurol. 1997; 244: 182-185.

348. Mohr DC, Goodkin DE, Likosky W et al. Treatment of depression improves adherence to interferon beta-1b therapy for multiple sclerosis. Arc Neurol 1997; 54:531-533.

349. Moller A, Wiedemann G, Rohde U, Backmund H, Sonntag A. Correlates of cognitive impairment and depressive mood disorder in multiple sclerosis. Acta Psy-chiatr Scand 1994; 89: 117-121.

350.Monge Argiles JA, Palacios Ortega F, Vila Sobrino JA, Matías-Guiu J. Heart rate variability in multiple sclerosis during a stable phase. Acta Neurol Scand 1998; 97: 86-92

351. Monod J. El azar y la necesidad. Ensayo sobre la filosofía natural de la biología moderna. Seix Barral, Barcelona 1971.

352. Monteyne P, Bureau JF, Brahic M. The infection of mouse by Theiler's virus: from genetics to immunology. Immunol Rev 1997; 159: 163-176

353. Montgomery RD. HTLV-1 and tropical spastic paraparesis. 1. Clinical features, pathology and epidemiology. Trans R Soc Trop Med Hyg 1989; 83:724-728.

354. Moore GRW. Neuropathology and pathophysiology of the multiple sclerosis lesion. En: Paty DW, Ebers GC. Multiple sclerosis, pp 257-327. FA Davis Company, Philadelphia 1998

355. Moore PM, Lisak RP. Multiple sclerosis and Sjogren's syndrome: a problem in diagnosis or in definition of two disorders of unknown etiology? (editorial). Ann Neurol 1990; 27:585-586.

356. Morgagni GB. De sedibus et causis morborum (1761). Citado en Porter (1997).

357. Morris JC. Case of the late Dr CW Pennock. Am J med Sci 1868; 56:138-144 (citado por DeJong 1970).

358. Morselt AF. The role of environmental factors and pollutants in combination with genetic predisposition in the etiology of multiple sclerosis: possibilities for prevention? (letter). J Child Neurol 1989; 4:228-229.

359. Moscarello MA, Wood DD, Ackerley C, Boulias C. Myelin in multiple sclerosis is developmentally immature. J Clin Invest 1994; 94:146-154.

360. Moulin DE, Foley KM, Ebers GC. Pain syndromes in multiple sclerosis. Neurology 1988; 38:1830-1834.

361. Moxon D. Case of insular sclerosis of brain and spinal cord. Lancet 1873; 1:236.

362. Mueller ME, Gruenthal M, Olson WL, Olson WH. Gabapentin for relief of upper motor neuron symptoms in multiple sclerosis. Arch Phys Med Rehabil 1997; 78:521-524.

363. Muller FA, Hanny PE, Wichman W et al. Cerebrospinal fluid immunoglobulins and multiple sclerosis. Arch Neurol 1989; 46: 367-371.

364. Munschauer III FE, Kinkel RP. Managing side effects of interferon-beta in patients with relapsin-remitting multiple sclerosis. Clinical Therapeutics 1997; 19:883-893.

365. Murrell TGC, Hasrbige LS, Robinson IC. A review of the aetiology of multiple sclerosis: an ecological approach. Ann Hum Biol 1991; 18: 95-112.

366. Myhr KM, Riise T, Barrett-Connor E, Myrmel H, Vedeler C, Gronning M, Kalvenes MB, Nyland H. Altered antibody pattern to Epstein-Barr virus but not to other herpesviruses in multiple sclerosis: a population based case-control study from western Norway. J Neurol Neurosurg Psychiatry 1998; 64: 539-542

367. Nadol JB Jr. Vestibular neuritis. Otolaryngol Head Neck Surg 1995; 112:162-72.

368. Nelson DA. Dorsal root ganglia may be reservoirs of viral infection in multiple sclerosis. Med Hypotheses 1993; 40:278-283.

369. Nelson LM, Franklin GM, Jones MC. Risk of multiple sclerosis exacerbation during pregnancy and breast-feeding. JAMA 1988; 259:3441-3443.

370. Nicoletti R, Mina A, Balzaretti G, Tessera G, Ghezzi A. Transito intestinale con marker radiopachi nei pazienti affetti da sclerosi multipla. Radiol Med (Torino) 1992; 83:428-430.

371. Niedner H. Mitología nórdica. Edicomunicación, Barcelona 1997.

372. Nielsen L, Larsen AM, Munk M, Vestergaard BF. Human herpesvirus-6 immunoglobulin G antibodies in patients with   multiple sclerosis. Acta Neurol Scand Suppl 1997; 169:76-78.

373. Nimzowitch A. Mi sistema. Ricardo Aguilera Editor, Madrid 1971.

374. Noronha A, Toscas A, Jensen MA. Contrasting effects of alpha, beta and gamma interferons on nonspecific suppressor function in multiple sclerosis. Ann Neurol 1992; 31: 103-106.

375. Noseworthy JH, Miller DH. Measurement of treatment efficacy and new trial results in multiple sclerosis. Current Opinion in Neurology 1997; 10:201-210.

376. Noy S, Achiron A, Gabbay U, Barak Y, Rotstein Z, Laor N, Sarova-Pinhas I. A new approach to affective symptoms in relapsing-remitting multiple sclerosis. Compr Psychiatry 1995; 36: 390-395.

377. Oger JJF, Vorobeychick G, Al-Fahim A, Aziz T, Edan G, Paty D. Neutralizing antibodies in Betaseron-treated MS patients and in vitro immune function before treatment. Neurology 1997; 48: A80.

378. Oksenberg JR, Hauser SL. New insights into the immunogenetics of multiple sclerosis. Current Opinion in Neurology 1997; 10:181-185.

379. O'Neil D, Byrne E, Roberts L, Gates P. Hemitonic seizures: etiological and diagnostic considerations. Acta Neurol Scand 1991; 84:59-64.

380. Operskalski EA, Visscher BR, Malmgren RM, Detels R. A case-control study of multiple sclerosis. Neurology 1989; 39:825-829.
381. Ordia JI, Fischer E, Adamski E, Spatz EL. Chronic intrathecal delivery of baclofen by a programmable pump for the treatment of severe spasticity. J Neurosurg 1996; 85:452-457.

382. O'Riordan JI. Central nervous system white matter diseases other than multiple sclerosis. Current Opinion in Neurology 1997; 10:211-214.

383. Orn P. [Is UV radiation the explana-tion of geographical distribution? A new theory on latitude differences in the occurrence of multiple sclerosis]. UV-stralning forklarar geografisk spridning? Ny teori om latitudskillnaderna i utbredningen av multipel skleros. Lakartidningen 1998; 95: 825

384. Ortega y Gasset J. Para una psicología del hombre interesante. Revista de Occidente, XXV (julio 1925). En: Ortega y Gasset J. Para la cultura del amor. Ediciones El arquero, Madrid 1988.

385. Pachmann L. Estrategia moderna en ajedrez. Ediciones Martínez Roca, Barcelona 1971.

386. Page RI. Mitos nórdicos. Akal, Madrid 1992.

387. Panitch HS, Hirsch RL, Haley AS, Johnson KP. Exacerbations of multiple sclerosis in patients treated with gamma interferon. Lancet 1987; 1: 893-895.

388. Papo T, Marcellin P, Bernuau J, Durand F, Poynard T, Benhamou JP. Autoimmune chronic hepatitis exacerbated by alpha-interferon. Ann Intern Med 1992; 116:51-53.

389. Paris C. El animal cultural. Biología y cultura en la realidad humana. Ed. Crítica, Barcelona 1994.

390. Paty DW. The interferon-beta 1b clinical trial and its implications for other trials. Ann Neurol 1994; 36 (suppl): S113-114.

391. Paty DW, Ebers GC. Multiple sclerosis. FA Davis Company, Philadelphia 1998 (*passim*).

392. Paty DW, Hashimoto SA, Ebers GC. Management of multiple sclerosis and interpretation of clinical trials. En: Paty DW, Ebers GC (eds). Multiple sclerosis, pp 427-545. FA Davis Company, Philadelphia 1998.

393. Paty DW, Li DKB, UBC MS/MRI Study Group, and the IFNB Multiple Sclerosis Study Group. Interferon beta-1b is effective in relpssing-remitting multiple sclerosis. II. MRI analysis results of a multicenter, randomized, double-blind, placebo-controlled trial. Neurology 1993; 43:662-667.

394. Pellkofer M, Paulig M. Vergleichende Doppelblindstudie zur Wirksamkeit und Ver-traglichkeit von Baclofen, Tetrazepam und Ti-zanidin bei spastischer Bewegungsstorung der unteren Extremitaten. Med Klin 1989; 84:5-8.

395. Pellegrino R, Roberts A, Harper-Bennie J. The use of in-home portable conductive cooling units. Multiple Sclerosis Association of America, Cherry Hill, NJ 1997.

396. Peña Yáñez A, Suárez Pañeda JR, González Maldonado R, Morata Pérez J, Vela Bueno A. Sistematización de las narcolepsias en modelos estructurales: el síndrome de Pickwick como variante. Rev Neurología 1977; 24:355-370.

397. Peraire M. Diagnostico y tratamiento del paciente con neuralgia del trigémino. Neurologia 1997; 12: 12-22.

398. Pestka S. The purification and manufacture of human interferons. Sci Amer 1983; 249: 36-43.

399. Phadke JG. Survival pattern and cause of death in patients with multiple sclerosis: results from an epidemiological survey in north east Scotland. J Neurol Neurosurg Psychiatry 1987; 50:523-531.

400. Phadke JG. Clinical aspects of multiple sclerosis in north-east Scotland with particular reference to its course and prognosis. Brain 1990; 113:1597-1628.

401. Phadke JG, Downie AW. Epidemilogy of multiple sclerosis in the north-east (Grampian region) of Scotland -an update. J Epidemiol Community Health 1987; 41: 5-13.

402. Piscane A, Impagliazzo N, Russo M et al. Breast feeding and multiple sclerosis. Br Med J 1994; 308: 1411-1412.

403. Platón. Las leyes, o Sobre la legislación (hacia 357-347 aC), II, 653d. Centro de Estudios Constitucionales, 1983.*

404. Pliskin NH, Hamer DP, Goldstein DS et al. Improved delayed visual reproduction test performance in MS patients receiving interferon beta-1b. Neurology 1996; 47: 1463-1468.

405. Pliskin NH, Towle VL, Hamer DP et al. The effects of interferon-beta on cognitive function in multiple sclerosis. Ann Neurol 1994; 36:326.

406. Plohmann AM, Kappos-L, Ammann W, Thordai A, Wittwer A, Huber S, Bellaiche Y, Lechner-Scott J. Computer assisted retraining of attentional impairments in patients with multiple sclerosis. J Neurol Neurosurg Psychiatry 1998; 64: 455-462

407. Portenoy RK, Yang K, Thorton D. Chronic intractable pain: an atypical presentation of multiple sclerosis. J Neurol 1988; 235:226-228.

408. Porter R. The greatest benefit to mankind. A medical history of humanity from antiquity to the present. Harper Collins Pub, London 1997.

409. Poser CM. Multiple sclerosis. Observations and reflections--a personal memoir. J Neurol Sci 1992; 107: 127-140.

410. Poser CM. The epidemiology of multiple sclerosis: a general overview. Ann Neurol 1994; 36 (suppl): 180-193.

411. Poser CM. The dissemination of multiple sclerosis: a Viking saga? A historical essay. Ann Neurol 1994; 36 (suppl 2):S231-243. (b)
412. Poser CM. Viking voyages: the origin of multiple sclerosis? An essay in medical history. Acta Neurol Scand 1995 (suppl); 161: 11-22.

413. Poser CM. Notes on the epidemiology of multiple sclerosis. J Formos Med Assoc 1995; 94:300-308. (b)

414. Poser S, Kurtzke JF, Poser W, Schlaf G. Survival in multiple sclerosis. J Clin Epidemiol 1989; 42:159-168.

415. Poser CM, Paty DW, Scheinberg L, McDonald WI, Davis FA, Ebers GC, Johnson KP, Sibley WA, Silberberg DH, Tourtellotte WW. New diagnostic criteria for multiple sclerosis: guidelines for research protocols. Ann Neurol 1983; 13:227-231.

416. Pozzilli C, Bastianello S, Padovani A et al. Anterior corpus callosum atrophy and verbal fluency in multiple sclerosis. Cortex 1991; 27: 441-445. (a)

417. Pozzilli C, Fieschi C, Perani D, Paulesu E, Comi G. Relationship between corpus callosum atrophy and cerebral metabolic assymmetries in multiple sclerosis. J Neurol Sci 1992; 112: 51-57.

418. Pozzilli C, Gasperini C, Anzini A, Grasso MG, Ristori G, Fieschi C. Anatomical and functional correlates of cognitive deficit in multiple sclerosis. J Neurol Sci 1993; 115 (suppl):S55-8.
419. Pozzilli C, Passafiume D, Bernardi S, Pantano P, Incoccia C, Bastianello S, Bozzao L, Lenzi GL, Fieschi C. SPECT, MRI and cognitive functions in multiple sclerosis. J Neurol Neurosurg Psychiatry 1991; 54:110-115.(b)

420. Povey R, Dowie R, Prett G. Learning to live with multiple sclerosis. Sheldom Press, London 1997.

421. Prada A. Se canta lo que se pierde. Fonomusic 1980.

422. Proust M. A la recherche du temps perdu (1913). Alianza Editorial, Madrid 1975.*

423. Pryse-Phillips W. Companion to Clinical Neurology. Little, Brown and Co, Boston 1995.

424. Pryse-Phillips WE. The incidence and prevalence of multiple sclerosis in Newfoundland and Labrador, 1960-1984. Ann Neurol 1986; 20: 323-328.

425. Pugnetti L, Mendozzi L, Motta A et al. MRI and cognitive patterns in relapsing remitting multiple sclerosis. J Neurol Sci 1993; 115 (suppl):59-65.

426. Quevedo y Villegas F (1580-1645). Poesía original completa. Planeta, Barcelona 1981.

427. Rao SM. Neuropsychology of multiple sclerosis: A critical review. J Clin Exp Neuropsychol 1986; 8:503-542.

428. Rao SM. Neuropsychology of multiple sclerosis. Curr Opin Neurol 1995; 8: 216-220.

429. Rao SM, Hammeke TA, McQuillen MP et al. Memory disturbances in chronic progressive multiple sclerosis. Arch Neurol 1984; 41: 625.

430. Rao SM, Leo GJ, Bernardin L et al. Cognitive dysfunction in multiple sclerosis, I. Frecuency, patterns, and predictions. Neurology 1991; 41: 685-690.

431. Rao SM, Leo GJ, Ellington L, Nauertz T, Bernardin L, Unverzagt F. Cognitive dysfunction in multiple sclerosis, II. Impact on employment   and social functioning. Neurology 1991; 41: 692-696.

432. Reid TR. El imperio romano. National Geographic 1997, 1:2-41.

433. Reingold SC. Advances in the understanding and treatment of multiple sclerosis. J Neuroimmunol 1993; 44:221-224.

434. Revilla F. Diccionario de iconografía y simbología. Ed. Cátedra, Madrid 1995.

435. Reynolds EH. Multiple sclerosis and vitamin B12 metabolism. J Neuroimmunol 1992; 40: 225-230.

436. Riikonen R. The role of infection and vaccination in the genesis of optic neuritis and multiple sclerosis in children. Acta Neurol Scand 1989; 80:425-431.

437. Riise T, Gronning M, Aarli JA, Nyland H, Larsen JP, Edland A. Prognostic factors for life expectancy in multiple sclerosis analysed by Cox-models. J Clin Epidemiol 1988; 41:1031-1036.

438. Ritchie Russell W. Multiple sclerosis: occupation and social group at onset. Lancet 1971; ii: 832-834.

439. Rohowsky-Kochan C, Dowling PC, Cook SD. Canine distemper virus-specific antibodies in multiple sclerosis. Neurology 1995; 45:1554-1560.

440. Rolak LA. Multiple sclerosis. En: Evans R (ed). Prognosis of neurological disorders, pp 295-300. Oxford University Press, New York 1992.

441. Rolak LA. Neurology secrets. Hanley & Belfus Inc, Philadelphia 1993.

442. Roman GC. Retrovirus-associated myelopathies. Arch Neurol 1987; 44:659-663.

443. Roman GC, Schoenberg BS, Madden DL, Sever JL, Hugon J, Ludolph A, Spencer PS. Human T-lymphotropic virus type I antibodies in the serum of patients with tropical spastic paraparesis in the Seychelles. Arch Neurol 1987; 44:605-607.

444. Ron MA, Callanan MM, Warrington EK. Cognitive anomalies in multiple sclerosis: a psychometric and MRI study. Psychol Med 1991; 21:59-68.

445. Roquer J, Vallecillo G, Palomeras E, Pou A. Manifestaciones paroxísticas en la esclerosis múltiple. Neurología 1997; 12: 369-370.

446. Rosati G. Descriptive epidemiology of multiple sclerosis in Europe in the 1980s: a critical overview. Ann Neurol 1994; 36 (suppl): 164-174.

447. Rosati G, Aiello I, Pirastru MI, Mannu L, Sanna G, Sau GF, Sotgiu S. Epidemiology of multiple sclerosis in Northwestern Sardinia: further evidence for higuer frecuency in Sardinians compared to other Italians. Neuroepidemiology 1996; 15: 10-19.

448. Rose AS, Kuzuma JW, Kurtzke JF, Namerow NS, Sibley WA, Tourtellotte WW. Cooperative study in the evaluation of therapy in multiple sclerosis: ACTH vs. Placebo. Neurology 1970; 20:1-59.

449. Ross RT, Cheang M. Common infectious diseases in a population with low multiple sclerosis and varicella occurrence. J Clin Epidemiol 1997; 50: 337-339.

450. Ross RT, Nicolle LE, Cheang M. Varicella zoster virus and multiple sclerosis in a Hutterite population. J Clin Epidemiol 1995; 48: 1319-1324.

451. Ross RT, Nicolle LE, Dawood MR, Cheang M, Feschuk C. Varicella zoster antibodies after herpes zoster, varicella and multiple sclerosis. Can J Neurol Sci 1997; 24: 137-139.

452. Rothwell PM, McDowell Z, Wong CK, Dorman PJ. Doctors and patients don't agree: cross sectional study of patients' and doctors' perceptions and assessments of disability in multiple sclerosis. BMJ 1997; 314: 1580-1583.

453. Rudge P. J Neurol Neurosurg Psychiatry 1991; 54: 853-855 (citado por Barraquer-Bordás).

454. Rudick RA, Sibley W, Durelli L. Treatment of multiple sclerosis with type I interferons. En: Goodkin DE, Rudick RA. Multiple sclerosis. Advances in clinical trial design, treatment and future perspectives. Springer, London 1996.

455. Rumpf HJ, Wessel K. [Coping pattern and adjustment in multiple sclerosis] Copingmuster und Adaptivitat bei multipler Sklerose. Nervenarzt 1995; 66: 624-629.

456. Runmarker B, Andersen O. Pregnancy is associated with a lower risk of onset and a better prognosis in multiple sclerosis. Brain 1995; 118:253-261.

457. Sabatini U, Pozzilli C, Pantano P, Koudriavtseva T, Padovani A, Millefiorini E, Di Biasi C, Gualdi GF, Salvetti M, Lenzi GL. Involvement of the limbic system in multiple sclerosis patients with depressive disorders. Biol Psychiatry 1996; 39: 970-975.

458. Sadovnick AD. Genetic epidemiology of multiple sclerosis: a survey. Ann Neurol 1994; 36 (Suppl 2P):S194-203.

459. Sadovnick AD, Bulman D, Ebers GC. Parent-child concordance in multiple sclerosis. Ann Neurol 1991; 29:252-255.

460. Sadovnick AD, Ebers GC. Epidemiology of multiple sclerosis: a critical overview. Can J Neurol Sci 1993; 20: 17-29.

461. Sandyk R. Rapid normalization of visual evoked potentials by picoTesla range magnetic fields in chronic progressive multiple sclerosis. Int J Neurosci 1994; 77:243-59.

462. Sandyk R. Premenstrual exacerbation of symptoms in multiple sclerosis is attenuated by treatment with weak electromagnetic fields. Int J Neurosci 1995; 83:187-198. (a)

463. Sandyk R. Weak electromagnetic fields restore dream recall in patients with multiple sclerosis. Int J Neurosci 1995; 82: 113-125. (b)

464. Sandyk R. The pineal gland, cataplexy, and multiple sclerosis. Int J Neurosci 1995; 83:153-163. (c)

465. Sandyk R. Long term beneficial effects of weak electromagnetic fields in multiple sclerosis. Int J Neurosci 1995; 83:45-57.(d)

466. Sandyk R. Treatment with electromagnetic field alters the clinical course of chronic progressive multiple sclerosis -a case report. Int J Neurosci 1996; 88:75-82.

467. Sandyk R, Awerbuch GI. The pineal gland in multiple sclerosis. Int J Neurosci 1991; 61:61-67.

468. Sandyk R, Awerbuch GI.Vitamin B12 and its relationship to age of onset of multiple sclerosis. Int J Neurosci 1993; 71:93-99. (a)

469. Sandyk R, Awerbuch GI.Nocturnal melatonin secretion in suicidal patients with multiple sclerosis. Int J Neurosci 1993; 71:173-182.(b)

470. Sau GF, Aiello I, Siracusano S, Belgrano M, Pastorino M, Balsamo P, Magnano I, Rosati G. Pudendal nerve somatosensory evoked potentials in probable multiple sclerosis. Ital J Neurol Sci 1997; 18: 289-291

471. Saul RF, Hayat G, Selhorst JB. Visual evoked potentials during hyperthermia. J Neuroophthalmol 1995; 15:70-78.
472. Savettieri G, Elian M, Giordano D, Grimaldi G, Ventura A, Dean G. A further study on the prevalence of multiple sclerosis in Sicily: Caltanissetta city. Acta Neurol Scand. 1986 Jan. 73(1). P 71-5.

473. Savettieri G, Salemi G, Ragonese P, Aridon P, Scola G, Randisi G. Prevalence and incidence of multiple sclerosis in the city of Monreale, Italy. J Neurol. 1998; 245: 40-43

474. Sayetta RB. Theories of the etiology of multiple sclerosis: a critical review. J Clin Lab Immunol 1986; 21:55-70.

475. Schiffer RB, Weitkamp LR, Wineman NM, Guttormsen S. Multiple sclerosis and affective disorder. Family History, sex, and HLA-DR antigens. Arch Neurol 1988; 45:1345-1348.

476. Schluter B, Aguigah G, Andler W. Hypersomnie bei Multipler Sklerose. Klin Padiatr 1996; 208:103-105.

477. Schubert DS; Foliart RH. Increased depression in multiple sclerosis patients. A meta-analysis. Psychosomatics 1993; 34:124-130.

478. Schwartz GG. Multiple sclerosis and prostate cancer: what do their similar geographies suggest? Neuroepidemiology 1992; 11:244-254.

479. Scolding N. Strategies for repair and remyelination in demyelinating diseases. Current Opinion in Neurology 1997; 10:193-200.

480. Scott TF. Diseases that mimic multiple sclerosis. Postgrad Med 1991; 89:187-191.

481. Seguin EC, Shaw JC, van Derveer A. A contribution to the pathological anatomy of disseminated cerebro-spinal sclerosis. J Nerv Ment Dis 1878; 5:281-293 (citado por DeJong 1970).

482. Sehlen S, Uhlenbrock D. MR-Untersuchungen zur Geschlechts-, Alters- und Krankheitsabhangigkeit der Eisen-ablagerungen im Gehirn. Digitale Bild-diagn 1988; 8:70-77.

483. Selhorst JB, Saul RF. Uhthoff and his symptom. J Neuroophthalmol 1995; 15: 63-69.

484. Sellal F. Les demences sous-corticales. Rev Med Interne 1996; 17:419-424.

485. Sepcic J, Mesaros E, Materljan E, Sepic-Grahovac D. Nutritional factors and multiple sclerosis in Gorski Kotar, Croatia. Neuroepidemiology 1993; 12:234-240.

486. Shapira K, Poskanzer DC, Newell DJ, Miller HD. Marriage, pregnancy and multiple sclerosis. Brain 1966; 89: 419-428.

487. Sharief MK, Thompson EJ. Intrathecal immunoglobulin M synthesis in multiple sclerosis. Relationship with clinical and cerebrospinal fluid parameters. Brain 1991; 114:181-195.

488. Shepherd DI, Summers A. Prevalence of multiple sclerosis in Rochdale. J Neurol Neurosurg Psychiatry 1996; 61:415-417.

489. Siblerud RL. A comparison of mental health of multiple sclerosis patients with silver/mercury dental fillings and those with fillings removed. Psychol Rep 1992; 70: 1139-1151.

490. Sibley WA. Therapeutic claims in multiple sclerosis. Demos Vermande, New York 1996. (*passim*)

491. Sibley WA, Bamford CR, Clark K. Clinical viral infections and multiple sclerosis. Lancet 1985; i: 1313-1315.

492. Sinclair HM. Deficiency of essential fatty acids and atherosclerosis etcetera. Lancet 1956; 1: 381-383.

493. Skegg DC, Corwin PA, Craven RS, Malloch JA, Pollock M. Occurrence of multiple sclerosis in the north and south of New Zealand. J Neurol Neurosurg Psychiatry 1987; 50:134-139.

494. Sloan JB, Berk MA, Gebel HM, Fretzin DF. Multiple sclerosis and systemic lupus erythematosus. Occurrence in two generations of the same family. Arch Intern Med 1987; 147:1317-1320.

495. Smith AS, Meisler DM, Weinstein MA, Tomsak RL, Hanson MR, Rudick RA, Farris BK, Ransohoff RM. High-signal periventricular lesions in patients with sarcoidosis: neurosarcoidosis or multiple sclerosis? AJR Am J Roentgenol 1989; 153:147-152.

496. Smith CR, Shapiro RT. Neurology. En: Kalb RC (ed). Multiple sclerosis. The questions you have, the answers you need, pp 7-39. Demos Vermande, New York 1996.

497. Sobel RA. Anatomía patológica de la esclerosis múltiple. En: Antel JP. Esclerosis múltiple. Clínicas Neurológicas de Norteamérica, 1995; 1:1-21.

498. Sola P, Merelli E, Marasca R et al. Human herpesvirus 6 and multiple sclerosis: survey of anti-HHV-6 antibodies by immunofluorescence analysis and of viral sequences by polymerase chain reaction. J Neurol Neurosurg Psychiatry 1993; 56: 917-919.

499. Sorensen PS. Intravenous immuno-globulin G therapy: effects of acute and chronic treatment in multiple sclerosis. Mult Scler 1996; 1: 349-352

500. Souberbielle BE, Martin-Mondiere C, O'Brien ME, Carydakis C, Cesaro P, Degos JD. A case-control epidemiological study of MS in the Paris area with particular reference to past disease history and profession.Acta Neurol Scand 1990; 82:303-310.

501. Stackpoole A, Mertin J. The effect of prostaglandin precursos in *in vivo* models of cell mediated immunity. Prog Lipid Res 1981; 20: 649-654.

502. Staerman F, Coeurdacier P, Guiraud P, Cipolla B, Lobel B. Valeur diagnostique de l'enregistrement des erections nocturnes. Prog Urol 1996; 6:403-408.

503. Stenager E, Knudsen L, Jensen K. Acute and chronic pain syndromes in multiple sclerosis. Acta Neurol Scand 1991; 84:197-200.

504. Stenager E, Stenager EN, Jensen K. Multiple sclerosis and sex. Semin Neurol 1992; 12: 120-124.

505. Stenager E, Stenager EN, Jensen K. Sexual function in multiple sclerosis. A 5-year follow-up study. Ital J Neurol Sci 1996; 17:67-69.

506. Stevenson RL. El club de los suicidas (1880). Unidad Editorial, Madrid 1998.*

507. Stip E, Truelle JL. Syndrome de personnalite organique dans la sclerose en plaque et influence du stress sur les poussées. Can J Psychiatry 1994; 39: 27-33.

508. Storch M, Lassmann H. Pathology and pathogenesis of demyelinating diseases. Current Opinion in Neurology 1997; 10:186-192.

509. Swank RL. Multiple sclerosis: a correlation of its incidence with dietary fat. Am J Med Sci 1950; 220: 421-430.

510. Swank RL. Multiple sclerosis: fat-oil relationship. Nutrition 1991; 7:368-376.

511. Swank RL, Grimsgaard A. Multiple sclerosis: the lipid relationship. Am J Clin Nutr 1988; 48:1387-1393.

512. Swank RL, Lerstead O, Strom A, Backer J. Multiple sclerosis in rural Norway. N Engl J Med 1952; 246: 721-728.

513. Symons AL, Bortolanza M, Godden S, Seymour G. A preliminary study into the dental health status of multiple sclerosis patients. Spec Care Dentist 1993; 13:96-101.

514. Taggart HM. Multiple sclerosis update. Orthop Nurs 1998; 17: 23-27.

515. Tan CT. Prognosis of patients who present with an episode of myelopathy of unknown origin in Malaysia: a retrospective study of 52 patients. Aust N Z J Med 1989; 19:297-302.

516. Tanaka M, Suzuki T, Endo K, Harayama H. [A case of multiple sclerosis with galactorrhea amenorrhea syndrome]. Rinsho Shinkeigaku 1997; 37: 483-486.

517. The Canadian Cooperative Multiple Sclerosis Study Group. The Canadian cooperative trial of cyclophosphamide and plasma exchange in progressive multiple sclerosis. Lancet 1991; 337:441-446.

518. Theiler M. Spontaneous encepahlo-myelitis of mice: A new virus disease. Science 1934; 80:122.

519. Thompson AJ, Noseworthy JH. New treatments for multiple sclerosis: a clinical perspective. Current Opinion in Neurology 1996; 39: 187-198.

520. Tienari PJ.Multiple sclerosis: multiple etiologies, multiple genes? Ann Med 1994; 26:259-269.

521. Trapp BD, Peterson J, Ransohoff RM, Rudick R, Mork S, Bo L. Axonal transection in the lesions of multiple sclerosis. N Engl J Med 1998; 338: 278-285.

522. Traynelis VC, Hitchon PW, Yuh WT, Kaufman HH. Magnetic resonance imaging and posttraumatic Lhermitte's sign. J Spinal Disord 1990; 3:376-379.

523. Trotot PM, Cabanis EA, Lavayssiere R, Sansonetti PJ, Sandoz-Tronca C, Cabee AE, Tamraz J, Stoffels C, Levillain PM. Apport de l'IRM cerebrale a l'etude des facteurs pronostiques du SIDA. Hypotheses a partir de l'examen de 15 patients. J Radiol 1988; 69:193-196.

524. Trotot PM, Sansonetti PJ, Levillain R, Cabanis EA, Lavayssiere R, Sandoz-Tronca C. Imagerie par resonance magnetique: depistage precoce des atteintes du systeme nerveux central au cours du syndrome d'immuno-deficience acquise (SIDA). C R Acad Sci III 1988; 307:1-4.

525. Tsunoda I, Fujinami RS. Two models for multiple sclerosis: experimental allergic encephalomyelitis and Theiler's murine encephalomyelitis virus. J Neuropathol Exp Neurol 1996; 55:673-686.

526. Uede T, Nonaka T, Takigami M, Fujishige M, Tanabe S, Hashi K. [Cavernous malformation of the brain stem: clinical symptom and its surgical indication]. No Shinkei Geka 1991; 19:27-34.

527. Uldry PA, Regli F, Uske A. Apport de l'imagerie par resonance magnetique dans les atteintes medullaires: 127 cas. Schweiz Rundsch Med Prax 1992; 81:1048-1054.

528. Uria DF, Calatayud MT, Virgala P, Díaz A, Chamizo C, Dean G. Multiple sclerosis in Gijon health district, Asturias, northern Spain. Acta Neurol Scand 1997; 96: 375-379

529. Uria DF, Virgala P, Alonso P, Crespo JR, Calatayud T, Arribas JM. Epidemiologia de la esclerosis multiple en Asturias. Neurología 1991; 6:41-45.

530. Vahtera T, Haaranen M, Viramo Koskela AL, Ruutiainen J. Pelvic floor rehabilitation is effective in patients with multiple sclerosis. Clin Rehabil 1997; 11: 211-219.

531. Valberg LS, Flanagan PR, Kertesz A, Ebers GC. Abnormalities in iron metabolism in multiple sclerosis. Can J Neurol Sci 1989; 16:184-186.

532. van Waesberghe JH, Castelijns J, Barkhof F. Magnetization transfer imaging in multiple sclerosis. Int MSJ 1996; 3: 47-57.

533. Vassallo L, Elian M, Dean G. Multiple sclerosis in Southern Europe. II: Prevalence in Malta in 1978. J Epidemiol Comm Health 1979; 33: 11-13.

534. Vercoulen JH, Hommes OR, Swanink CM, Jongen PJ, Fennis JF, Galama JM, van der Meer JW, Bleijenberg G. The measurement of fatigue in patients with multiple sclerosis. A multidimensional comparison with patients with chronic fatigue syndrome and healthy subjects. Arch Neurol 1996; 53:642-649.

535. Verdier-Taillefer MH, Alperovitch A. Do male patients with multiple sclerosis have an excess of female offspring? Neuroepidemiology 1991; 10:18-23.

536. Visscher BR, Clark VA, Detels R et al. Two populations with multiple sclerosis. Clinical and demographic characteristics. J Neurol 1981; 225: 237-249.

537. Voskuhl RR, Pitchekian-Halabi H, MacKenzie-Graham A, McFarland HF, Raine CS. Gender differences in autoimmune demyelination in the mouse: implications for multiple sclerosis. Ann Neurol 1996; 39:724-733.

538. Walsh A, Walsh PA. Love, self-esteem, and multiple sclerosis. Soc Sci Med 1989; 29: 793-798.

539. Walters ML. Chronic sorrow in multiple sclerosis: a case study (letter). Home Healthc Nurse 1994; 12:57.

540. Warnell P. The pain experience of a multiple sclerosis population: a descriptive study. Axone 1991; 13:26-28.

541. Warner HB, Carp RI. Multiple sclerosis etiology -an Epstein-Barr virus hypothesis. Med Hypotheses 1988; 25:93-97.

542. Warren SA, Warren KG, Greenhill S, Paterson M. How multiple sclerosis is related to animal illness, stress and diabetes? Can Med Assoc J 1982; 126: 377-385.

543. Warren S; Warren KG; Cockerill R. Emotional stress and coping in multiple sclerosis (MS) exacerbations. J Psychosom Res 1991; 35:37-47.

544. Watanabe I, Iijima H, Imai M. Recovery of visual field defects in ischemic optic neuropathy and idiopathic optic neuritis]. Nippon Ganka Gakkai Zasshi 1991; 95:986-994.

545. Weinreb HJ. Multiple sclerosis (1995-1996). http://aspin .asu.edu/ msnews/ weinreb1.htm

546. Weinshenker BG. Epidemiology of multiple sclerosis. Neurol Clin 1996; 14:291-308.

547. Wellingham-Jones P. Characteristics of handwriting of subjects with multiple sclerosis. Percept Mot Skills 1991; 73: 867-879.

548. Wheeler G, Krausher K, Cumming C, Jung V, Steadward R, Cumming D. Personal styles and ways of coping in individuals who use wheelchairs.AADE Ed J 1996; 34:351-357.

549. Whitham RH, Bourdette DN. Treatment of multiple sclerosis with high-dose methylprednisolone pulse therapy. Neurology (suppl 1) 1989; 39:357. ***

550. Whitman W. Hojas de hierba. Orbis, Barcelona 1997.

551. Whittle IR, Hooper J, Pentland B. Thalamic deep brain stimulation for movement disorders due to multiple sclerosis [letter]. Lancet 1998; 351: 109-110.

552. Wiart L, Joseph PA, Petit H, Dosque JP, de Seze M, Brochet B, Deminiere C, Ferriere JM, Mazaux JM, N'Guyen P, Barat M. The effects of capsaicin on the neurogenic hyperreflexic detrusor. A double blind placebo controlled study in patients with spinal cord disease. Preliminary results. Spinal Cord 1998; 36: 95-99

553. Wild KV, Lezak MD, Whitham RH et al. Psychosocial impact of cognitive impariment in the multiple sclerosis patient. J Clin Exp Neuropsychol 1991; 13:74.

554. Wilhelm H, Grodd W, Schiefer U, Zrenner E. Uncommon chiasmal lesions: demyelinating disease, vasculitis, and cobalamin deficiency. Ger J Ophthalmol 1993; 2:234-240.

555. Williams KC, Ulvestad E, Hickey WF. Immunology of multiple sclerosis. Clin Neurosci 1994; 2:229-245.

556. Wojtowicz S. Multiple sclerosis and prions. Med Hypotheses 1993; 40:48-54.

557. Wynn DR; Rodriguez M; O'Fallon WM; Kurland LT. A reappraisal of the epidemiology of multiple sclerosis in Olmsted County, Minnesota. Neurology 1990; 40:780-786.

558. Yalaz K, Anlar B, Oktem F et al. Intraventricular interferon and oral inosiplex in the treatment of subacute sclerosing panencephalitis. Neurology 1992; 42: 488.

559. Yetkin FZ, Haughton VM, Papke RA, Fischer ME, Rao SM. Multiple sclerosis: specificity of MR for diagnosis. Radiology 1991; 178:447-451.

560. Yu YL, Woo E, Hawkins BR, Ho HC, Huang CY. Multiple sclerosis amongst Chinese in Hong Kong. Brain 1989; 112:1445-1467.

561. Zainqui JM. Diccionario razonado de sinónimos y contrarios. De Vecchi, Barcelona 1984.

562. Zeldow PB, Pavlou M. Physical and psychosocial functioning in multiple sclerosis: descriptions, correlations, and a tentative typology. Br J Med Psychol 1988; 61:185-195.

563. Zeman AZ, Keir G, Luxton R, Thompson EJ. Serum oligoclonal IgG is a common and persistent finding in multiple sclerosis, and has a systemic source. QJM 1996; 89:187-193.

564. Zilber N, Kahana E. Risk factors for multiple sclerosis: a case-control study in Israel. Acta Neurol Scand 1996; 94: 395-403.

FOOTNOTES BY CHAPTERS

PROLOGUE - FOOTNOTE

*Prof. Eduardo Varela de Seijas is one of Spain´s greatest neurologists, having taught innumerable colleagues of mine at his Service at the Hospital Clínico de Madrid. His scientific knowledge, in continuous renewal, is supported by an immense and diverse body of cultural knowledge, and his broad conception of the world brings to mind the full extent of meaning of "the humanities." He also has the great defect of excessive benevolence prologuing friends. Gracias, Eduardo.

INTRO - FOOTNOTE

*A hot bath can trigger or aggravate symptoms in multiple sclerosis patients.

CHAPTER 1 - FOOTNOTES

Eponym means *"The one that gives his/her name."* In ancient times, the word eponym was used to designate the person (normally a magistrate or priest) who gave the city its name for a year and was mentioned in decrees. This honor came at a price, and in times of scarce resources, nobody wished to take on the eponymy. In such a case, it was assigned to a god. For instance, during hard times in Miletus, Apollo was designated eponym.[145]

*Besides being a great philosopher, Baltasar Gracián was a good Jesuit. To brainy males tempted by the evils of the flesh, he advised discretion: *"Reputation consists more of reserve than of deed, and if one is not chaste, so should he be cautious,"* he wrote (inspired by the old Latin saying, *Sis castior, dodalis, aut sis cautior*).[186]

*"Oligodendrocytes" is a word made up of Greek terms: *oligos*=pequeño, *dendros*=prolongation, ramification, and *cytos*=cell. That is, "cells with small prolongations."

***Open the bodies and you will see the disease,"** said Morgagni (1682-1771) in his book *De sedibus et causis morborum ("Of the Locations and Causes of Disease")*. It is the defining principle of Anatomical Pathology: the causes of an illness are traced to lesions in the body.

*According to Freud,[166] in hysteria there is a content of psychic representations that at some point has grown enough to take over the somatic innervation. He distinguishes between the motor phenomena of the hysterical crisis and the permanent symptoms. "Exacerbations" and "sequelae" are seen in hysteria as well.

**"Protean" means varied, with many forms or facies. Proteus was a god of the sea and the symbol of versatility, because he could alter his form at will. In the passage where he tries to escape from Menelaus, he changed into lion, snake, panther, boar, running water and tree.[191]

*Sir Francis Walshe noticed that multiple sclerosis patients were similar precisely insofar as their differences were concerned, with varying symptoms and evolutions: they share an *"air of unity in their variety."*

*Margulis, Soloviev and Shubladze (1948), cited by Barraquer.[28]

**The Champs de l'Elysèes are, in Greek mythology, the equivalent of the Christian Paris, the Muslim Eden, or the Viking Valhalla: humans believe that good souls should be awarded (as angels, houris, or valkyries) when they die.

*Heinrich Heine is not only known for his songs to castles, witches, gnomes and Gothic temples. He was a revolutionary burger and an incredulous Voltarian. His verse and prose reveal a mixture of irony, sarcasm and skepticism.

*The description is offered by J.C. Morris on December 4, 1867, in his conference to the College of Physicians of Philadelphia, titled: "The Case of the Late Dr. C.W. Pennock."

**Profusus*, in Latin, means "extensive spill." *Ecumenical* means "universal" (from the Greek *oikumènè* = occupied land); it is a very useful term that should not be limited to religious references.

*This is from Quevedo: [426] "With just a few good books gathered together (...), if not always understood, always open at least, to enrich or straighten out my affairs" (*Con pocos pero doctos libros juntos (...) si no siempre entendidos, siempre abiertos, o enmiendan o fecundan mis asuntos"*).

CHAPTER 2 - FOOTNOTES

*The **grey matter** (cerebral cortex, nuclei of nerve cells and the inner core of the spinal cord)contains the bodies of the neurons with their dendrites (the short branches). The **white substance** is the area crossed by the long axons, forming ascending (sensitive) pathways or descending (motor) pathways.

*This heading is structured after the famous phrase *Delenda est Cartago* ("May Carthage be destroyed"), which was uttered by the Roman statesman Cato the Elder (234-149 B.C.) at the end of each speech he made before the consuls of Rome. These were the times of the Punic Wars, and Cato was determined to foment a hatred of Carthaginians.

*Galen (c.130-c.200) defined the **thymus** as "the gland of valor and affection." *Thymus* means "affection"; therefore, a person with "dys-thymia" is one who has trouble organizing his or her emotions. In reality, the thymus has important immunological functions, particularly in early life.

**Other autoimmune diseases are rheumatoid arthritis and myasthenia, in which the cartilage or the neuromuscular synapses of the organism are damaged.

*"Acerbate" (from acerb = acid) means to aggravate or exasperate), whereas "acervate" (*adj*) means growing in heaps or clusters.[70,96]

**The blood-brain barrier (BBB)is a concept: the anatomical and physiological structures that come between the blood and the brain act as filters. Under normal conditions, they have a "selective" permeability, impeding the passage of certain substances and cells. When the barrier is "broken" as a result of a traumatism or some other cause, elements normally unable to enter the brain may do so.

*The Phoenix is a symbol of what appears to be dead but may come to life again (like chronic plaques, like some loves). In Egyptian mythology, the phoenix is a great bird, appearing gray while buried in its ashes, then resurrecting as an eagle with gold and crimson wings.[128]

*There are other congenital diseases with metabolic disorders that cause myelin damage (e.g. metachromatic leukodystrophy, adrenal leukodystrophy, leukodystrophy), but their evolution is different, being chronic and with symptoms present since infancy.

*Sixty drachmas per year were the wages of the Greek heralds. They were to announce the peace settlements or the honors in dionysian feasts, and stood out in cultural ceremonies (Aristotle was a herald of Athens for ten years).[145] Herald came to mean "messenger," the one who announces an upcoming event such as a ceremony or the arrival of a prince.[96,561]

*To be more specific, one would have to reach the jungle known as "Semliki"; hence the name "Semliki Forest virus."

CHAPTER 3 - FOOTNOTES

*The legendary team of law enforcement agents nicknamed The Untouchables was headed by Eliot Ness.

*Sardinia was invaded by Phoenician, Roman, Byzantine, Genoese, and Spanish ships, among others. Its inhabitants learned to look toward the sea with fear in their hearts, and repeat the old Sardinian saying "*Chi venit da'e su mare furat* ("He who comes from the sea is a plunderer.")

**When Hercules went to hunt the lion of Citheron, he spent fifty days at the residence of King Thespis, who was determined to have descendants of the hero. Each night Hercules was invited to sleep with one of the fifty daughters of the King, and Hercules, at the ardent age of eighteen, left all but one of them pregnant (she later became a virgin priestess). As the eldest and the youngest of the daughters both had twins, the grandchildren of Thespis (The Thespidians) numbered 51, though only 40 of them colonized Sardinia.

*The initials **HLA** (Human Leukocyte Antigen) designate molecules that are key to our immunological system. There are two types (HLA I and II). **MHC** (Major Histocompatibility Complex) designates another type of substance that is decisive for the normal immune response.

Promiscuity means a mixture or tendency to mix (in excess). It comes from Latin: *pro-* = tendency to, *miscere* = to mix. This word is often misused with sexual connotations (perhaps because persons who spend too much time together end up getting involved?).

*The Viking language was similar to what was then spoken by Germans, Dutch and Anglo-Saxons. In some islands of the North Atlantic the original Viking language is still spoken today, and might be understood by someone familiar with English: for instance, *Ég er víkingur frá Íslandi* would be "*I am a Viking from Iceland.*"

**The article[412] is titled "Viking voyages: the origin of multiple sclerosis? An essay in medical history."

***Christopher Columbus did not discover America. Five centuries earlier, Eric the Red and his crew went from Iceland to Greenland, which is not so surprising if we take a good look at a map or globe: only about one thousand kilometers separate Europe and North America at that point.

*Odin is the main god of Viking mythology. Curiously enough, Norse gods were mortal, unlike their Greek or Roman counterparts.[371,386]

**The Hutterites, or Hutterian Brethren, are a Mennonite sect founded by Jakob Hutter (c.1500 - 1536), a Tyrolean Anabaptist. The study referred to consisted of 5,601 clinical histories, and the serum antibodies to herpes zoster-varicella of 315 Hutterites and 259 control subjects of other religious backgrounds.[449-450]

*There are some exceptions to the predominance among women: some Carpathian communities[62] have equal incidence in the two sexes, and among Turkocypriots there are more men than women with multiple sclerosis.[102]

*In France, more girls than boys are born each year (1.05:1 ratio). According to a broad survey (8,000 patients of both sexes), among French women with multiple sclerosis, birthrate is even higher than the overall average. [535]

*A study of 15,815 same-sex pairs of twins showed coincidence of the disease in two of the seven monozygotic pairs, and none of the dizygotic twins.[257]

**The "family" risk of suffering from multiple sclerosis varies with the age at onset of symptoms: in patients under 20, 8.9% of the siblings will be affected; between age 21 and 30, risk drops to 5.1%, and continues to decline from 31 to 40 years of age (3.1%), 41 to 50 (1.3%) and is minimal — reversed, in fact— after age 50 (0.6%).[459]

CHAPTER 4 - FOOTNOTES

*When Phaëton lost control of the horses that pulled the "golden chariot" of his father (Helios/Apollo), the course of the Sun was changed: at some points it was distanced from the Earth, forming the gelid poles, whereas at other points it got too close, creating desert areas. **Ovid** narrates the episode in his *Metamorphoses: "They approach the Earth... And such destruction is done! Trees, fields, cities and men are charred! Every mountain is an Etna in eruption! (...) The Nile retreated to the ends of the world. (...) From this fiery adventure, it is said, Ethiopia was left brown, and Libya, barren.*

*The Faeroe or Faröe Islands are located in the North Atlantic Ocean, northeast of Great Britain. In the 9th century they were invaded by Norwegians, and since 1380 they belong to the Danish crown. At the beginning of World War II they were occupied by the British before the German Naval forces could get there.

*Mercury is also used in instruments of measurement (thermometers or barometers) because, though a metal, it is liquid. This mobility gives it its name: Mercury had wings on his feet, and was the god of travel and commerce.

***Licht, mehr Licht*! ("Light, more light!") were the words pronounced by Goethe just before he died on March 22, 1832.

*I always avoid the expression "and/or" (an overused loan from Logic). Here it is used with sarcasm, as an excuse to cite Spanish linguist Lázaro Carreter:[289] "If this nonsense progresses, we must prepare ourselves to attend teas at which the hostess asks, "Would you care for coffee and/or milk?"

**A number of viruses are under suspicion: measles, rabies, herpes simplex, parainfluenza viruses, scrapie, *Paramyxovirus, Coronavirus,* monkey B virus, HTLV-1. The human herpesvirus 6 was a top suspect for a time, but serum antibodies (IgG) in different states showed no difference with controls in a 1997 study.[372]

*Neurotropic (*neuro* = nervous, and *tropos* = affinity) means having a predilection for the nervous system.

*English readers are no doubt familiar with the Encyclopedia Britannica, yet they may not know that Jorge Luis Borges read it from the very first to the very last page.

**"Bird on the Wire" is one of Leonard Cohen´s best known songs.

*"Chance and necessity" is the title of a well-known essay by Jacques Monod[351] about the causality and casuality of events.

*A prion is a miniscule protein particle with an infective capacity; it is distinguished from a virus in that it does not have intrinsic nucleic acids. In "classic" prion diseases ("mad cow" disease, kuru, scrapie), prions affect neurons, whereas, according to this hypotheses, in multiple sclerosis, the oligodendrocytes would be affected.

*The original metaphor refers to the disease that some call love: *Tus ojos y los míos se han enredado, como las zarzamoras en los vallados* ("Your eyes and mine are tangled up, like blackberry brambles on a fence"). From a poem by Miguel Hernández.

CHAPTER 5 – FOOTNOTES

**Avant-la lettre* is a French loan that means "in advance." Originally it was used to refer to the printer´s proofs of a picture that was not yet accompanied by an inscription or wording of any sort. These first copies, made with a "fresh" new plate, were the highest appraised.[223]

*The lesion may even affect bilaterally the medial longitudinal fasciculus producing an internuclear ophtalmoplegia; the patient sees double when looking to the right, and when looking to the left, but retains convergence (for example, can read well). If this occurs in a young adult, it is almost sure to be a case of multiple sclerosis.

**Medullary (spinal cord) reflexes are autonomous, though not completely so, as they can be controlled or interrupted by superior segments of the CNS such as the neurons of the cerebral cortex (which has a pyramidal form); it sends its orders via axons that descend to the spinal cord, thus constituting the pathway of the pyramidal tract.

*Papal bull is an edict of pardon. It was a document relieving an individual of a specific obligation that the Pope sealed with his leaden stamp called the *bulla.*

CHAPTER 6 - FOOTNOTES

*Confirmation of Charcot´s idea came a full century later:[259, 427] "*At some stage in the disease there is a noteworthy deterioration of memory, conceptualization is slow, and the intellectual and emotional faculties are dulled overall.*"[76]

*The capital of Laconia was war-plagued Sparta, where austerity reached such an extreme that the oratory (that decadent Athenian fashion) was prohibited. And so, nowadays, *laconic* describes a person who avoids conversation.

*Dementia is a medieval allegory representing "*a bedraggled man with a truncheon, walking amid stones probably thrown at him by children, imitating the cruel custom of stoning madmen.*"[434]

*Depression is variable, and there are methodological difficulties involved in its evaluation,[51] but statistical meta-analysis of six separate studies shows that it is very frequent among multiple sclerosis patients. [477]

*In reactions of stress or alert, the body releases cortisol (which increases cholesterol), as well as adrenaline and noradrenaline (two important neurotransmitters), making the pulse accelerate, the muscles tense, and the senses more acute.

**Stress and the social setting influence the appearance and the exacerbations of a number of neurological conditions: multiple sclerosis, epileptic crises, and cerebrovascular accidents.[188]

***Certain endogenous proteins[253] are produced, which may act as target antigens for the T lymphocytes.

*The personality or psychic structure of a person (just like his/her skeleton or eye color) may have a genetic base, not just from one´s parents, but from more distant ancestors as well (even from species preceding man) if we agree with Jung:[244] "According to the fundamental phylogenetic law, the psychic structure should, just as the anatomic one, carry within the prints of the ancestral grades crossed."

*Ortega y Gasset[384] deduces the psychology of an individual by the way he or she loves: "*In love, the condition and nature of the soul are reflected. If one is not very discerning, how is love to be clairvoyant? If one is shallow, how can his love be deep? As one is, so does he love.*"

*Amancio Prada is probably Spain's greatest singer/songwriter. In one of the warm gatherings at the home of Amalia, surrounded by friends, strawberries and nymphs, we left conversation unfinished when the morning glasses broke.

CHAPTER 7 - FOOTNOTES

* "*Sex, the scenography of the human unconscious, constitutes a space for drama and play by which to make present those areas of the memory that are scarcely accessible. We know, since Freud, that none of that which takes place in its display admits secular moral evaluation. Like any game, that of sex is governed only by the previous codification of rules among adults.*" (Gabriel Albiac)[6]

*So said Gowers: "Multiple sclerosis begins during gestation, remains stationary until the following pregnancy, and then becomes more progressive."

**A patient with incontinence may urinate with great frequency, though the total volume of urine may or may not also be great.

*The Lhermitte sign: when the patient flexes at the neck, a sensation of electric-like shocks (normally unpleasant) extends down the spine to the legs. It is observed in multiple sclerosis, and also in traumatisms or other pathologies involving the upper spinal cord.

**A symptom or sign is pathognomonic (from the Greek *pathos*=disease + *gnosis*=knowing) when its mere presence reveals a specific disease. For example, high glycemia is pathognomonic for diabetes (except under very special circumstances).

***When the discriminating Romans took baths, it was either in a *Caldarium* (hot bath), *Tepidarium* (tepid bath), or *Frigidarium* (cold bath). They also had a sort of swimming pool where the temperature was not controlled, the *Natatio.* This distribution can be seen in the Thermal Baths of Caracalla, in Rome.[432]

*Wilhelm Uthoff was a well-known neuro-ophthalmologist, possibly the first clinician to dedicate his life to this subspecialty halfway between the fields of Neurology and Opthalmology.

*This verse is from Antonio Enrique,[17] friend and poet of extraordinary sensitivity. It reminds me of what patients with hysteria or multiple sclerosis might say using simpler words: *Te nace una zarza entre las ingles / un alacrán y espigas locas crecen en mi pecho* ("Brambles take root around your groin/ a scorpion and spikes of wild grain grow in my chest").

*There are isolated descriptions of crises of tonic extension of all the members owing to a contralateral lesion of the brain stem.[297]

*Our heart beats and our breathing comes automatically, even when we are not aware. In mythology, Ondine was condemned to carry out all such automatic functions in a voluntary mode; that is why a sleep disorder with associated disturbances of spontaneous breathing (and other problems with the neurovegetative system) is known as *Ondine's curse.*

CHAPTER 8 - FOOTNOTES

*Diagnosis comes from the Greek (*dia*=separate + *gnosis*=knowing). Although some dissatisfied patients might prefer the definition by Ambrose Bierce (*The Devil's Dictionary*, 1906):[53] *Diagnosis: prognosis of disease made by a doctor who takes the patient's pulse and purse.*

*The time elapsing between the first symptoms and the diagnosis is getting shorter and shorter. One recent Italian study, for instance, estimated the interval at five years, while in the 80's in that same area the diagnosis took some nine years.[473]

**The oligoclonal bands of immunoglobulin G (IgG) are obtained by electrophoresis. They are quite specific for multiple sclerosis, though they can be seen in other inflammatory processes such as syphilis, menigoencephalitis, and polyradiculoneuritis.[441] The IgG index has a sensitivity of 63% and specificity of 65%, and the probability of a positive result is 1.80 (2.40 without corticoids). [299]

**In half of patients the immunoglobulin G is also increased in serum, suggesting a systemic immunological disturbance, not one limited to the nerve tissue.[563]

*The hot water test produces symptoms because the demylinated nerves are very sensitive to heat. This can be objectively assessed in the visual evoked potentials: when the temperature rises more than one degree, the amplitude of the P2 wave diminishes. [471]

*Our classic poet Quevedo (1580-1645)[426] describes impotence in the context of old age: *La boca despoblada por los años, las potencias, de ejercicio ajenas...* ("One's mouth left uninhabited by the years, one's powers exercised by a force beyond").

*In Latin, *pudendus* means *"which cause shame."*

**Out of 29 impotent MS patients, 26 showed alterations in the evoked potentials of the pudendal nerve; the other three were cases of psychological etiology.[258]

***A well-known verse by Zorilla (1817-1893): *A buen juez, mejor testigo* ("For a good judge, an even better witness").

*It is an "off-resonance" technique of contrast by irradiation of the tisular reservoir of protons bound to immobile macromolecules; it produces an effect of lost signals between the different tissues which is very marked in the brain. It can be adapted to conventional resonance equipment with no need for new hardware.

**The lesions are characterized by measuring the rate of magnetic transference, which indicates the degree to which the macromolecular matrix of a tissue is destroyed.

*Retroviruses infect vertebrates, and share some common elements with their genome; they produce neurological diseases with complex interactions between the viral antigen, the neurotoxic peptides that produce the virus, and the active cellular genes they induce. [192]

**HTLV-1 is the human virus of the T lymphocytes, a retrovirus associated with certain chronic neurological diseases. There is also another variety that produces a lymphoma/leukemia of T cells.

*The rate of infection is high: 1%-2% of the total population,[185] though of these, only 0.25% present spastic paralysis. Frequency depends on the mode of contagion, whether through mother's milk, blood transfusion, or sexual intercourse.[193]

CHAPTER 9 - FOOTNOTES

*Chronology is the study of events over time. It comes from the Greek; *cronos* means time and also represents *Cronus*, the god of time (equated with the Roman god Saturn). Among other deeds,

Cronus castrated his father, Uranus, and tried to destroy his children by devouring them (as seen in the famous painting by Goya).

*If one reaches adolescence without having had contact with this external factor, no harm will come even if there is a genetic predisposition.

**Myelin is necessary for the proper conservation of axons. If it suffers much damage, the axons will eventually undergo irreversible deterioration.

*In resonance imaging, the progressive forms have more infratentorial lesions with a greater tendency to coalesce.[261] The forms that are progressive from the onset show fewer inflammatory lesions (three per year) than the secondary progressive forms of MS (18 lesions per year, as seen using gadolinium). However, once progressive -whether primary or secondary- the clinical deterioration is similar.

*In over 80% of cases the first symptoms appear between the ages of 20 and 50; 7% before age 20; and 12% after age 50.[400] In Spain, the onset tends to come at around 29 years of age.[16, 233]

*A person from Spain with nasal congestion would say he is *constipado*; this is a false friend of the English "constipated." The two terms do share a Latin root, however: *constipar* means "to close or obstruct" physiological conducts, be they nasal or intestinal.[96]

**Not observing any symptoms does not necessarily mean that the disease will not be reactivated. A study now underway should throw some light on this distinction: magnetic resonance of vaccinated patients will reveal plaques that might not have produced symptoms.

*The lesions are very heterogeneous inter-individually (different from one patient to the next), but not intra-individually (similar within a single patient).

**There are four subgroups,[508] depending on the predominating type of lesion: 1) primary demyelination with little damage to oligodendrocytes; 2) demyelnation with a great loss of oligodenrdrocytes; 3) primary damage to oligodendrocytes and secondary demyelination; and 4) intense activation of macrophages that produce a non-selective destruction of myelin, oligodendrocytes, axons and astrocytes. These may possibly represent four forms of multiple sclerosis.

Collage is a French word (from *coller*=to paste) that is most often used to designate a variety of elements that are arranged in disorderly fashion. It became a pictorial technique in the hands of Braque, Picasso and Max Ernst (around 1912), and is considered basic to Dada and Surrealism. It consists of cutting natural or manufactured materials and pasting them on a surface where something suggested by the added element might be painted.

Suave mari magno relays the sense that it is agreeable for someone who has escaped the wide open sea to recall the dangers experienced. Lord Byron [65] evokes Lucretius with these words in his *Journal of Kefalonia*, inspired by a long overseas voyage, from Lisbon to Istanbul.

*Of 18 children with optic neuritis, ten had suffered a viral or bacterial infection in the two weeks previous, and six were affected after vaccination. Of those vaccinated, all but one developed multiple sclerosis later on. Of the post-infectious cases, five eventually developed multiple sclerosis.[436]

CHAPTER 10 - FOOTNOTES

Cuando me lo contaron sentí el frío / de una hoja de acero en las entrañas / me apoyé contra el muro, y un instante / la conciencia perdí de donde estaba... ("When they told me I felt the cold / of a steel blade in my entrails / I leant against the wall, and for a moment / I lost all sense of my surroundings...") These verses could describe what is felt by a patient just after hearing the neurologist's diagnosis. Yet in fact, they refer to the love sickness felt by Gustavo Adolfo Bécquer (1836-70).[41]

*The etymology of "strategy" takes us to the military vocabulary (*estrategos*, in Greek, is "general"). Here is a trick question that might trip up more than one pedantic intellectual: *What is the etymology of the word "etymology"?* The correct answer —with a condescending smile— is that *etimos* means origin, truth.

**Desideratum* (plural, *desiderata*) is something desired as essential.

*The *Moirai* (Roman *Parcae*) were the Fates, three old women –Clotho, Lachesis and Atropos—who controlled human destiny. They spun, measured and cut the web of life. Atropos, in charge of cutting, lent her name to *Atropa belladonna*, a plant with lethal effects from which atropine is obtained.[191,434]

Augurs were highly respected diviners of ancient Rome, who reported or interpreted *auguries*. From this same root we have the word *inauguration*, because it was customary to observe the auguries of any new locale.[70,96]

*When the Romans appointed a new magistrate, indications of his future success were sought by observing the flight and feeding of birds, known as the *auspices* (*avis*=bird, *specere*=to look).

*The three godesses offered either power (Hera or Juno), wisdom (Athena or Minerva) and love (Aphrodite or Venus). The choice was a difficult one, and the apple of discord gave way to the Trojan War. May the reader put himself in the place of Paris and choose just one –power, wisdom or love (aware that "to choose is to leave behind").

CHAPTER 11 - FOOTNOTES

*In the embryo, the suprarenal glands are (were) nerve tissue, a sort of ganglial group that emigrated and became independent. In the adult, these glands no longer have visible connections with the nervous system, yet they respond to stress by producing hormones.

**The area of the brain that produces ACTH is the hypothalamus. The hormone is released by neurons there which are more active in persons with multiple sclerosis.[126]

*The words spoken to Judas by Jesus at the Last Supper (St John 13:27).[243]

**The corticoids and ACTH have many beneficial effects on the body's immune response:[144] they reduce the presence of T lymphocytes, block interferon gamma, decrease IgG and prostaglandin E_2 and improve the blood-brain barrier, for example.

*The rabbits had experimental allergic encephalitis, a sort of "artificial" MS, produced by injecting myelin (see Chapter 2).

**The usual doses of corticoids are 0.25-1 mg per kilo of weight and day (therefore, some 20-80 mg for an adult).

*It would appear that the intravenous megadose produces immuno-modulating effects that are not observed with lower oral doses;[267] for one, there is a greater efficacy as a result of the reduction of T cells (CD4+), which are active in the demyelinating processes of both optic neuritis and multiple sclerosis.

CHAPTER 12 - FOOTNOTES

*Azathioprine is a derivative of mercaptopurine. It acts as a general immunosuppressant, on both a cellular level (lymphocytes) and a humoral level (antibodies). The higher the dose (2-3 mg/kg/day), the lower the leukocyte count (some are alarmed when there are 3,000 leukocytes/mm^3, while others risk going as low as 2,000).

**Human testing uses the "double blind" method: patients are divided at random into two groups, one receiving the drug assumed to have therapeutic benefits, and the others getting a placebo (an innocuous product made of sugar, starch, water, etc., with the same aspect as the real medication). In order to avoid psychosomatic interference in the body´s response, neither the patient nor the physician is informed as to which substance is taken.

CHAPTER 13 - FOOTNOTES

*Nearly all the cells of an organism can produce interferons, but most important are the leukocytes (specializing in interferon alpha) and the fibroblasts (interferon beta).

**Interferon type II (gamma) is produced by the lymphocytes and the "natural killer" cells; it increases the number of flare-ups because it amplifies the immune responses without halting the suppressant activity.[52,374,387]

*Of 372 patients with recurring multiple sclerosis, three groups were established by the administration of: subcutaneous placebo, low-dose interferon beta (1.6 MIU), and high dose (8 MIU). Two years later, the average number of flare-ups was determined, respectively, as 1.27, 1.17 and 0.83.

*Hermeneutics consist of interpreting the keys or hidden significance of something; in this case, it would be relating resonance images to their meaning.

*This phenomenon is also seen in diabetics with insulin injections: neutralizing antibodies are produced, thereby reducing the initial efficacy of treatment (above all in the days when pig or cow insulin was used).

**The patients with a more active form of the disease produce more neutralizing antibodies, and this might be predicted by the basal secretion rate of IgG.[377]

*Interferon gamma is elaborated by T lymphocytes in response to some specific antigens, is thought to be involved in the inflammatory reaction, activates the macrophages (which destroy myelin in these patients), alters the blood-brain barrier, and in addition, has been shown to aggravate the experimental model of MS.

*Aside from increasing the "natural killer" lymphocytes, linomide has other immuno-modulating and antiviral properties, and it can prevent experimental allergic encephalitis.

*Other growth factors are under study as well, such as those derived from platelets (PDGF) and from fibroblasts (FGF).

CHAPTER 14 - FOOTNOTES

*Baclofen relaxes certain mechanisms of the central nervous system. Its structure is similar to that of GABA (gamma-aminobutyric acid), a neurotransmitter that inhibits reflexes of the spinal cord. It can be administered with a intrathecal perfusion pump, an efficient method that shortens hospital stays.[381] If it is chronic, male patients suffer reversible loss of erection and ejaculation.[106]

*Gabapentin is a curious drug: it was designed as an anti-epileptic, yet at low dosage it can be used to treat very diverse pathological processes: essential tremor, Parkinson's disease, muscular spasms, restless leg syndrome, and diverse neuralgias, among others.

**The injections of phenol must be repeated every three to six months; in some cases it is preferable to sever the nerve.[218]

*The mechanism at work would be the opposite of anti-epileptic action, as it augments the capacity of the neuron to "shoot off, " and for this reason it must be used with caution to avoid the risk of convulsions.

*In a recent study [151] the patients treated with interferon beta 1-a showed, at the end of two years, a clear overall neuropsychological improvement in comparison with the placebo group. This was even more evident in the categories "memory/information processing" and "visuo-spatial capacity/execution."

*"Martingalas" (an ancient name of Spanish origin) are special undergarments designed with additional deposits.

CHAPTER 15 - FOOTNOTES

*Mentor was a character of the Odyssey who took care of Telemachus during the long voyage of his father (a chap by the name of Ulysses). Now, "mentor" means spiritual or intellectual guide, yet centuries ago it referred to one who taught grammar on a tutorial basis.

*"Of the terrible doubt of appearances" is the title of a poem by Walt Whitman, in *The Leaves of Grass.*

*The "quality of life" scales, in which the patient offers subjective data, are growing in use. They tend to give discrepant results with other tests, such as the Kurtzke Scale.

*Baltasar Gracián tells the anecdote of the emperor who overcame adverse circumstances: when Caesar arrived in Africa, just off the ship, he tripped and fell face down on the ground. Instead of feeling embarrassed, he made the very best of it by stating "I hereby take possession of this land!"

CHAPTER 16 - FOOTNOTES

*A phrase from Giradoux, as quoted by columnist Manuel Alcántara ("Ideal," 09/06/1998).

*To straighten something we use an **orthesis** (*ortho*=straight). A **prosthesis** is a fabricated substitute, an addition; it can also be used to denote the addition of a sound or syllable to a word (e.g., a prefix), or the lateral apse of a basilica.[145]

*Occurring when the eyes do not coordinate their movement properly, either due to a lesion of the oculomotor nerves, or to alterations in the cerebellum or brain stem.

*Computer programs can be "trained" to adapt to the phonetics of an individual (after just a few samples of speech). Once recognized, the voice is digitalized, so that the computer can operate or write via dictation.

*Culture is more than a grouping of customs. It is an extracorporeal world that articulates with our biology to constitute a *new reign of reality.*[389] Michel Foucalt[160] calls it "the death of man": the ultimate identity of our being is dissolved in the (cultural) framework that makes up human reality. Thus, the individual's loss is society's gain.

**The foremost system of communication is that of the mass media (press and television), with a central "sender" and many "receivers" (readers, viewers) who have no contact among themselves, no individual reciprocity. The telephone, displacing the mail as the second communication system, has reciprocity only between two points: from individual to individual, with no group involvement.

*"Remora" is an interesting –though little used— synonym for "hindrance" or "impediment." Remora are fish with suctorial discs on their fins, enabling them to adhere to ships and, allegedly, slow them down.

**The Muses, daughters of Zeus and Mnemosyne (memory), numbered seven, representing the liberal arts: Calliope (eloquence), Euterpe (music), Erato (love poetry), Polyhymnia (sacred poetry), Clio (history), Melpomene (tragedy), Thalia (comedy), Terpischore (dance) and Urania (astronomy).

***Apollo is the god of beauty and Medicine, whereas Dionysus represents wine, fertility and unbridled behavior.

****Il dolce far niente ("the sweetness of doing nothing") is an Italian saying originating in a text by Pliny the Younger (c.62-113).

CHAPTER 17 - FOOTNOTES

*A diet without essential fatty acids alters cell membranes, microcirculation and other mechanisms that favor sclerosis.[31] Animals with this dietary deficit produce abnormal phospholipids, have altered myelin,[492] and are more susceptible to experimental allergic encephalitis.[501]

**This plasmatic drop in linoleic acid has also been observed in other general acute diseases, for which reason it might be a secondary phenomenon.[80]

*Other studies (of very limited size) found no differences between bottle- and breast-fed babies.[50,73]

**There is a sociological branch of epidemiology that pays special attention to the conduct and relationships of different social groups.[303]

*Oatmeal is not beyond suspicion either. In regions where it is grown more widely, the rate of mortality from multiple sclerosis is higher.[284]

*"To toil the earth" is precisely the meaning of **Georgics**, from the Greek georgós (gê=earth + érgon=work).

**Bucolics comes from the Latin bucolucus (=pastoral), in turn from the Greek bukólos (=oxman). It came to mean anything related with herds and pastures.

CHAPTER 18 - FOOTNOTES

*Paracelsus' real name was Theophrastus Bombastus von Hohenheim. He was a Swiss physician and alchemist (1493-1541) who traveled widely, basically because he thrown out of so many circles. He rejected the classical medical theories of Galen, Hippocrates and Avicenna, and held that man is a microcosm integrating all the processes, rhythms and forces of nature.

*There is no crime more wicked than that of a mother who harms her own children in vengeance of the father who abandoned her. Medea killed her two children when Jason left her for Creusa.

*Anyone interested can consult Internet (http://www.2bcool.com) or contact: Life Enhancement Technologies, Inc. Their telephone number is (1-800)779-6953, with fax (560) 568-5909.

*My dear old friend does not wish to reveal his true identity. He is a clever, unorthodox and slightly devilish neurologist, whom we will nickname "Hyde."

*"I will surrender my body to the pleasures, / to the enjoyments one dreams of, / to the great daring of erotic desire, / to the lustful burning of my blood, / with no fear..." Verses by Cavafis that could define the Epicurean doctrine, which was not as perverse as many people think.

*The antibodies in cow colostrum are assimilated by baby calves, but it is improbable that a person would assimilate them, as they would decompose in the human stomach.

**A chimera is an illusion or fantasy. In mythology, the *chimera* was a creature with a lion's head, goat's body and dragon's tail. In botany, the *chimera* is a "monstrous" hybrid formation of different vegetable species, for example by grafting. If you want to plant an almond tree on your lawn, where the moisture would be detrimental for the almond trunk, graft the almond branches onto a plum tree trunk, which resists humidity. The tiny deformed leaves at the graft union are also known as *chimeras.*

*Superoxide dismutase (SOD) is a metallo-proteic enzyme that neutralizes the oxygen free radicals (superoxides) by combining with them.

CHAPTER 19 - FOOTNOTES

Kyrie eleison is an invocation to God's mercy uttered near the beginning of the mass. Its origin can be traced to the Greek *kýrie eléeson* ("Lord have mercy!").

*I mentioned Gmarc back in the Chapter 1. It is the pseudonym of a multiple sclerosis patient who is also a doctor. That double condition, together with his fine sense of irony and communicative skills, allows him to clearly relate situations he has experienced. His Internet address is: http://aspin.asu.edu

CHAPTER 20 - FOOTNOTES

*José María Peinado is Professor of Biochemistry at the School of Medicine of the University of Granada. He teaches and conducts research in basic fields of the nervous system. He is also a member of the "Instituto de Neurociencias," which he founded and formerly directed.

*Daniel Serrano is the Head of the Ophthalmology Service of the Hospital Clínico in Granada, Spain.

**Juan Andrés Burguera coordinates the Movement Disorder Unit of the Hospital La Fe in Valencia, Spain, and has published widely on urinary problems associated with multiple sclerosis.

*Miguel Guerrero is in charge of the Multiple Sclerosis Unit of the Neurology Service of the Hospital Clínico of Granada.

*José Luis Jiménez Bullejos (Psychiatry teaching unit, CS Virgen de las Nieves) is well-experienced in the psychological monitoring of multiple sclerosis patients.

*Luis Javier López del Val (Neurology Service, Hospital Clínico Universitario of Zaragoza, Spain) is familiar with the use of nerve stimulators in the central nervous system.

*Alfonso Castro (Neurology Service, Hospital Clínico of Santiago de Compostela) is Tenured Professor of Neurology at that city's University. He is one of the neurologists with the most direct, extensive and intensive experience in the undergraduate teaching of our specialty

www.ingramcontent.com/pod-product-compliance
Lightning Source LLC
Chambersburg PA
CBHW080338290526
45790CB00010B/3746